HERBAL TEAS SIMPLIFIED

REDUCE STRESS, IMPROVE SLEEP AND DIGESTION TO
ENHANCE IMMUNITY FOR A VIBRANT, HEALTHY LIFE

BRIAN TURNER

© **Copyright 2023 - All rights reserved.**

The content contained within this book may not be reproduced, duplicated or transmitted without direct written permission from the author or the publisher.

Under no circumstances will any blame or legal responsibility be held against the publisher, or author, for any damages, reparation, or monetary loss due to the information contained within this book, either directly or indirectly.

Legal Notice:

This book is copyright protected. It is only for personal use. You cannot amend, distribute, sell, use, quote or paraphrase any part, or the content within this book, without the consent of the author or publisher.

Disclaimer Notice:

Please note the information contained within this document is for educational and entertainment purposes only. All effort has been executed to present accurate, up to date, reliable, complete information. No warranties of any kind are declared or implied. Readers acknowledge that the author is not engaged in the rendering of legal, financial, medical or professional advice. The content within this book has been derived from various sources. Please consult a licensed professional before attempting any techniques outlined in this book.

By reading this document, the reader agrees that under no circumstances is the author responsible for any losses, direct or indirect, that are incurred as a result of the use of the information contained within this document, including, but not limited to, errors, omissions, or inaccuracies.

TABLE OF CONTENTS

Introduction — 5

1. THYME TO EXPLORE THE FUNDAMENTALS OF HERBAL TEA — 11
   - So... What Is Herbal Tea? — 12
   - Herbal Tea's Rich Heritage — 15
   - Introducing the Healing Properties of Herbal Teas — 19
   - Where to Find Quality and Affordable Ingredients — 20
   - Tips for Brewing the Perfect Tea — 26

2. BALANCE FOR A HOLISTIC APPROACH TO WELLNESS — 29
   - The Importance of Taking a Holistic Approach to Wellness — 31
   - An Introduction to Tea-Drinking Rituals — 34
   - Incorporating Meditation and Mindfulness With Tea Drinking — 39

3. A GUIDE TO SIPPING SAFELY AND MINIMIZING RISK — 43
   - Potential Risks of Herbal Teas to Consider — 44
   - A Guide to Responsible Herbal Tea Consumption — 48
   - When in Doubt, Talk to a Doctor — 49

4. BECOME CHAMOMILE CALM WITH STRESS-RELIEVING TEAS — 53
   - Understanding Stress and Anxiety — 54
   - A Guide to Nature's Calming Herbs — 60
   - Anxiety and Stress-Relief Tea Recipes — 63
   - Interactive Element — 80

5. EXPERIENCE VALERIAN DREAMS WITH SLEEP-INDUCING TEAS — 85
   - The Science of Sleep — 86
   - A Guide to Nature's Sleep Aids — 89

Sleep-Enhancing Tea Recipes	93
Interactive Element	109
6. DISCOVER GINGER'S ZING WITH DIGESTIVE HEALTH-BOOSTING TEAS	111
A Guide to Digestive Wellness	113
Nature's Herbal Digestive Aids	119
Digestive Health-Supporting Tea Recipes	122
Interactive Element	137
7. BOOST YOUR IMMUNITY WITH ECHINACEA ELIXIRS AND OTHER TEAS	139
The Science Behind Building a Strong Immune System	141
A Guide to Immune-Boosting Herbs	144
Immune-Boosting Tea Recipes	147
Interactive Element	163
8. ACHIEVE SAGE SERENITY AND WELLNESS WITH THESE FINAL TEAS	167
The Path to Holistic Wellness	169
A Guide to Wellness-Enhancing Herbs	173
Healthy Tea Recipes	175
Interactive Element	191
Conclusion	195
References	199
About the Author	217

INTRODUCTION

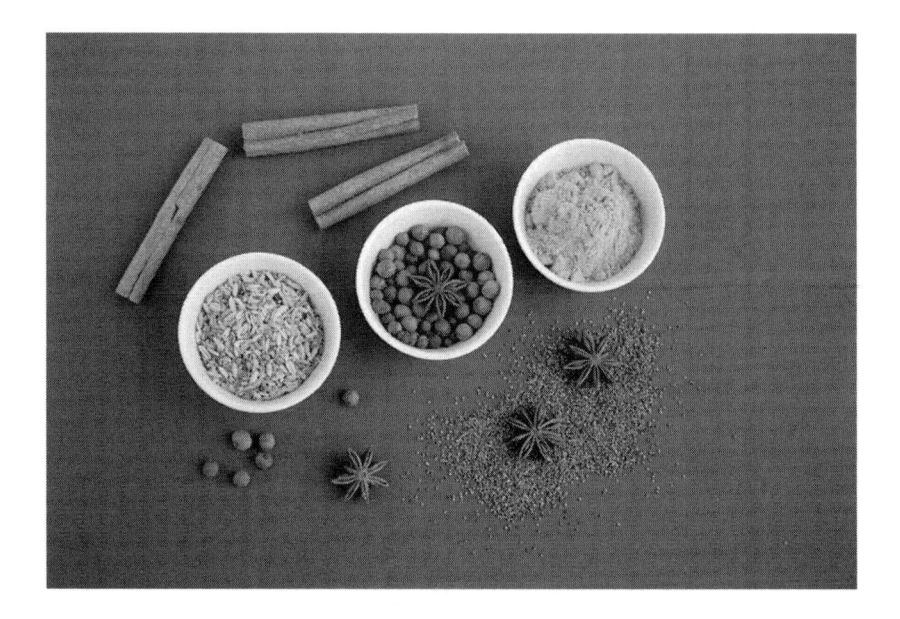

Can you imagine a life without depending on pharmaceuticals? What would that be like? Picture it: no more adverse reactions, no need to take this medication to counteract the effects of that medication, and no more insurance headaches. What if I told you I know of someone who did just that? Let's take a look at her story.

A woman named Heidi spent a significant portion of her life depending on the diagnoses and prescriptions of her physicians. Unfortunately, those prescriptions that were intended to make her better resulted in severe damage to her liver. The worst part was that her insurance wouldn't cover the bill to pay for the necessary treatment to mend the damage. Instead, she paid out of pocket, whittling away her and her husband's life savings.

To say the least, Heidi became pretty jaded with the whole conventional medicine practice. She asked herself those same what-if questions and came up with the ideal solution for her needs: herbalism. With all-natural products that she crafted herself, she took charge of her health and wellness journey, kicking conventional medicine to the curb.

Heidi planned and grew her own medicinal herb garden and practiced ethical and sustainable wildcrafting to source the most potent and healthy herbs for her needs. She spent a lot of her free time researching the best homemade remedies and found that herbal teas promised many significant benefits. With their versatility, she found she could customize each brew to meet her specific needs, whether it was to reduce the symptoms of the common cold, boost her immune system, or aid in digestive health. The best part about these remedies in her mind was that there was no significant risk to her health, unlike conventional medications.

Since then, Heidi and her husband have reduced their dependence on pharmaceuticals and very rarely visit their physician. In fact, with their boosted immunity, they rarely get sick now or need antibiotics. With the benefits of her herbal teas and other remedies, they have improved their overall health, saved money, and developed a sustainable way of living. She's also been able to turn her herbalism practice into a way to make money through teaching others (Villegas, 2023).

Today, many of us face lowered immunity, making us more susceptible to colds, infections, and generalized fatigue. On top of that, digestive problems are more common today than ever with the abundance of unhealthy foods available for everyone to eat. Because of these issues, herbal teas have an allure. You may be curious about the benefits you can gain, including increasing the variety of your diet with healthy drinks. Additionally, you may want to learn how to enrich your diet—even if it's top-notch—with high-quality drinks that will introduce potent vitamins, minerals, and antioxidants to boost your immune system and overall health and well-being.

It's all too common today for the average person to experience stress and anxiety. As a result, their sleep is often negatively impacted, leading to insomnia or poor sleep quality. While there are plenty of pharmaceutical options for sleep aids, these medications can potentially cause side effects, including addiction. Because of these potential complications, many individuals seek all-natural alternatives. Herbal teas can be formulated to help combat stress, anxiety, and sleep problems. You can formulate the ideal combination to target your specific needs, resulting in better overall health.

Within the pages of this book, I will present to you the concept of TEAS:

- **T** - Tea's healing properties, history, and fundamentals will be covered in Chapter 1.
- **E** - Essential tips for making a holistic and balanced approach to health and wellness will be discussed in Chapter 2.
- **A** - Applicable safety tips for risk-free herbal tea drinking will be presented in Chapter 3.
- **S** - Scrumptious tea recipes, tea-drinking rituals, herbal information, and much more will be presented in Chapters 4–8.

When presenting tea recipes, I'll offer several different types, including those to reduce stress and anxiety, enhance sleep, improve digestive health, boost your immunity, and promote overall wellness. Herbal teas are highly versatile and customizable, allowing you to create exactly what you need when you need it.

By the end of this book, you will have the knowledge you need to safely craft your own herbal teas to improve your health and wellness. From understanding what herbal teas are to how to take a holistic approach to your health and wellness, I'll provide the tools you need to successfully take charge of your healing with herbal teas.

I have spent significant time learning about herbal teas. From my personal experience, I can attest to the powerful remedies and healing they offer. Because I have found so many positive benefits from drinking herbal teas, I decided to write this book to share my knowledge with you. I understand how tricky it can be to navigate the world of herbalism without guidance, especially if it's your first journey into using medicinal plants.

Throughout history, herbs have been successfully used for healing many ailments. Because of their demonstrated efficacy, they are still widely used today in many cultures worldwide. However, finding exactly what you need in such a vast sea of information can be daunting, especially if you're someone who has never done more than purchase a box of chamomile tea from the store.

To make the process easier and more understandable, I will break it down piece by piece. The world of herbalism and herbal teas is at your fingertips and ready for you to take the plunge into optimizing your health and wellness with the highest quality products and no chemicals. You'll quickly be on your way to a holistic lifestyle.

To get started, it's essential to understand the fundamentals of herbal tea. In our first chapter together, we will explore all the crucial topics, including the heritage of herbal teas, where to source quality ingredients, and how herbal teas can benefit your health and wellness. Let's get started on our journey together.

10 | INTRODUCTION

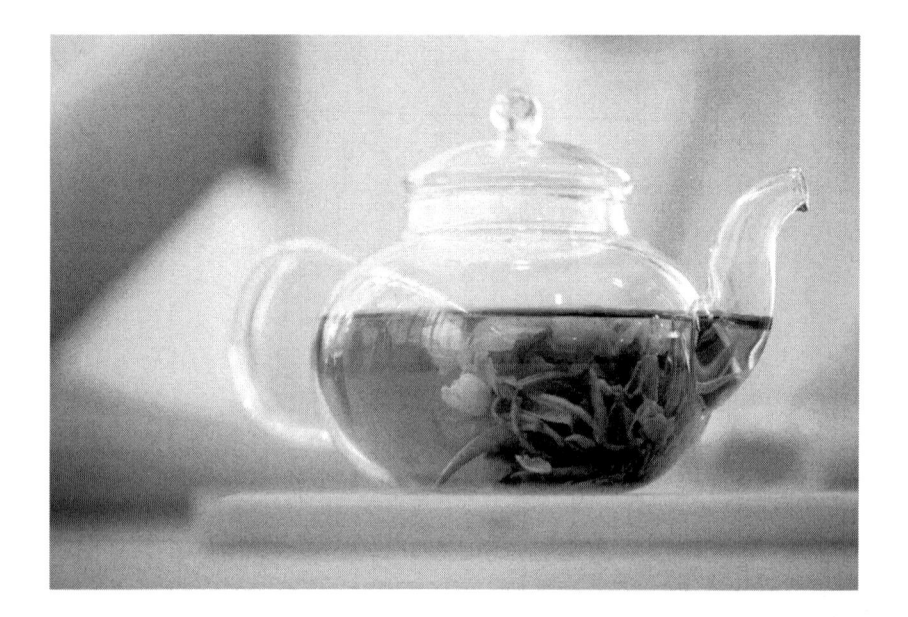

1

THYME TO EXPLORE THE FUNDAMENTALS OF HERBAL TEA

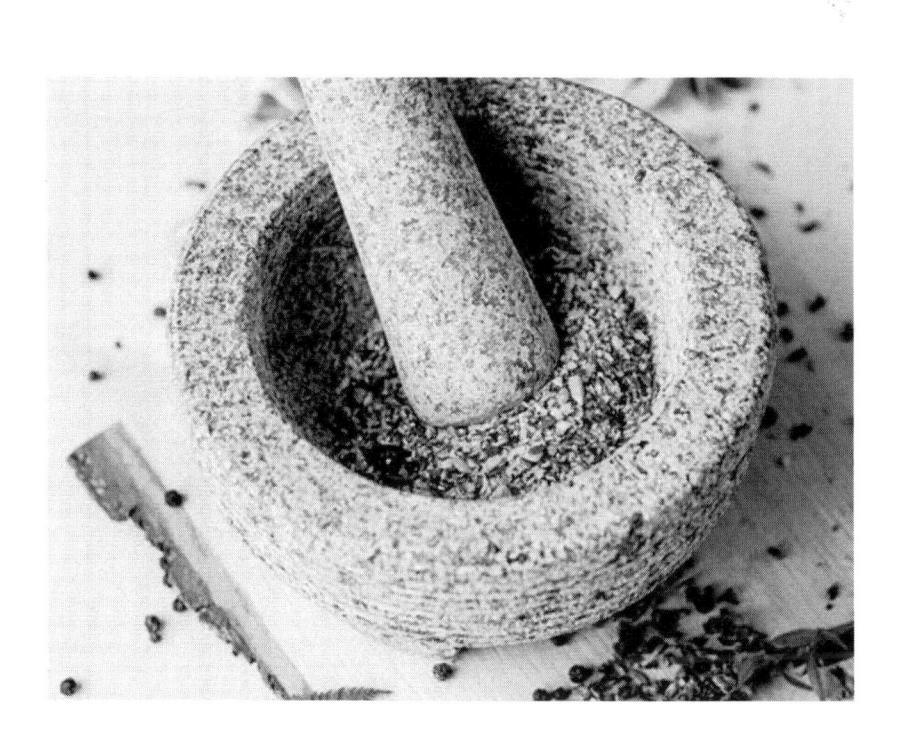

> *There is no problem on earth that can't be ameliorated by a hot bath and a cup of tea.*
>
> — JASPER FFORDE

Throughout history, many cultures have relied upon the power of herbs to heal and ease different ailments. One common method of administration is herbal tea. No matter what the condition, there has been an herbal tea recommended to address it.

These drinks have become increasingly popular in recent years as more individuals seek natural remedies to aid in their overall health and wellness journeys. Unfortunately, the herbal teas commercially available in the supermarket aren't always of the highest quality or even the real deal.

In this chapter, we'll explore the fundamentals of herbal tea, including how you can create your own herbal blends at home with high-quality ingredients. To get started, let's define what herbal tea is.

SO... WHAT IS HERBAL TEA?

While we call it *tea*, herbal tea is nothing of the sort. True teas are a derivative of the *Camellia sinensis* plant. These include the oolong, black, green, and white teas commonly consumed worldwide. Typically, these drinks have caffeine and are drunk as a regular beverage. For our purposes throughout this book, we'll be discussing herbal teas specifically.

Herbal teas are derived from edible plants. They're infusions or blends of various parts of these plants, including the leaves, flowers, fruits, bark, and roots. These drinks are more commonly known in Europe and various parts of the world as *tisanes*.

These beneficial drinks have become increasingly popular in recent years; however, they have a storied history that spans centuries. They have long been used to heal various ailments. Many cultures also believe herbal teas benefit the individual on a spiritual level.

Many common herbs are used in making herbal teas, including:

- chamomile
- ginger
- linden leaf
- holy basil
- fennel
- ginkgo biloba
- peppermint

Chamomile is well-known for its relaxing properties. It's beneficial for relieving insomnia when consumed before bed. Additionally, it can help reduce the effects of a sore stomach. For those with anxiety and stress, chamomile may have calming effects that reduce the symptoms.

Ginger has a long history of use as an anti-nausea agent. With its anti-inflammatory properties, it can reduce inflammation throughout the body. This inflammation can lead to several issues, including migraines and weight gain. Ginger is also known to reduce congestion and aid in reducing the effects of the common cold.

If you need to boost your immune system, consider linden leaf. Additionally, it functions like chamomile to reduce stress and anxiety. It also boasts anti-inflammatory properties, targeting inflammation that can cause a variety of ailments. One other perk is its ability to decrease the effects of a sore throat.

Holy basil has been widely used throughout history to treat various ailments, from bronchitis to malaria. It's good for the digestive tract, relieving upset stomach and preventing vomiting and diarrhea. This herb has also been used to prevent eye diseases, relieve congestion, and reduce fevers.

Fennel is an excellent herb for digestive support and appetite stimulation. Many have used it for the management of Crohn's disease, irritable bowel syndrome (IBS), and muscle spasms. Nursing mothers have often used it to stimulate milk production.

Ginkgo biloba is a great choice for stimulating blood circulation. This property allows it to help promote heart and mind health. It is an excellent tool for detoxing the body and easing the pain of headaches and cramps. It may also act as a natural mood stabilizer to aid those with depression and anxiety.

Peppermint is another reliable herb used for treating upset stomach, including IBS. It is also beneficial in the treatment of headaches and in reducing sinus pressure.

HERBAL TEA'S RICH HERITAGE

The use of herbal tea dates back to ancient times, including ancient Egyptian and ancient Chinese cultures. Texts have emerged from both cultures documenting their extensive use of herbal teas for medicinal advantages. They have also long been chosen in India as natural alternatives to traditional teas.

In the first century, Dioscorides, the well-known Greek physician, documented over 600 medicinal plants that could be steeped into herbal teas. On top of that, researchers of the Egyptian pyramids have found evidence of dried peppermint leaves dating back to 1000 B.C.E. They believe these herbs were used to aid digestion.

During the Middle Ages, monks and various followers of medical and alchemical schools transformed the preparation of herbal teas into a much more sophisticated process. They conducted many studies on medicinal herbs and broke them down into categories of effect and effectiveness.

Based on the information provided in historical records, these herbal teas were relied upon for medicinal purposes and their ability to invoke calmness and open the drinker to a greater sense of spiritual awareness. Eventually, many came to find the aromas and flavors pleasant, resulting in a much wider use of herbal teas.

Ancient Egypt

Herbal medicine played a significant role in ancient Egyptian culture. While health and wellness were perceived as a never-ending fight between the forces of good and evil, the physicians and magicians employed by the pharaohs constantly worked on developing medical care. Many complementary medicine modalities were developed during this period, including herbalism.

For their time, the physicians of Ancient Egypt were advanced in their practices. They had a basic understanding of human anatomy, including how the organs functioned, essentially due to the mummification practice employed upon the deaths of the pharaohs. Their pharmacy knowledge was equally impressive—these physicians had a broad range of knowledge about mixing herbal remedies.

Some of the herbal remedies used in Ancient Egypt included herbal teas. One in particular was coriander tea, which was taken to alleviate stomach and urinary problems. With the physicians' vast knowledge of herbalism, herbal teas were a common treatment option for various ailments.

China and Japan

Traditional Chinese medicine (TCM) has evolved over several centuries. One significant aspect of this school of thought is the practice of herbalism. TCM practitioners rely on herbal formulas to help boost the body's natural self-healing ability.

Herbal teas have a long history in the development of TCM and are largely believed to have been introduced during the Tang Dynasty. From there, they dramatically expanded in the Song Dynasty and finished maturing in the Qing Dynasty. Historical records have revealed at least eight types of herbal teas in the Qing Dynasty's emperor's medical files.

These teas were developed for the treatment of various conditions and ailments based on the properties of the herbs. As tea in general became increasingly popular, exports to Japan and other locations worldwide increased.

Japan also developed its traditional medical system, Kampo. While unique to the country's culture and practices, Kampo also relied on certain herbal teas to treat certain ailments and manage various chronic conditions.

India

According to Indian folklore, a king of the royal court had a tea-like drink concocted as a form of Ayurvedic medicine in ancient India. He wanted to provide healing solutions for his people and collected well-known healing ingredients. While it is unknown what the drink contained, it is speculated that the ingredients may have included ginger and black pepper for digestion, cardamom for mood, cloves for pain, cinnamon for circulation, and star anise for flavor. The mixture was served with warm water, almost like a tea (Worthington, 2020).

Undoubtedly, traditional teas have a large place in Indian culture. However, herbal teas are also very common, with Ayurvedic medicine having a solid cultural place in the country. Much like TCM, Ayurveda is practiced throughout the country, with herbal remedies relied upon for their numerous health benefits.

Ancient Africa

European settlers first introduced the practice of drinking tea to Africa in the 17th century. From there, the practice evolved into various indigenous plants as substitutes for both tea and coffee. However, vernacular names for teas were rarely recorded in the Khoi and San culinary traditions, indicating they were not part of the pre-colonial era before teas and coffees were introduced to the Cape. One of the more recently added Cape teas includes the popular rooibos tea. It's considered a newer invention, as it was absent from earlier literature, only making its presence known in the 19th century.

Ancient Greece and Rome

Ancient Greece and Rome used medical practices that relied heavily upon herbs and food as therapeutic tools. These cultures have a strong written history referencing the use of herbal remedies, including the Homeric epics and Homeric Hymns in the 8th century B.C.E. and the Hippocratic Corpus from around 450–350 B.C.E. Additionally, they have a rich oral history detailing the use of herbs. Historical artifacts in burial chambers and palaces support the use of plants in Greek culture.

Various herbal teas have been consumed since ancient times for their therapeutic benefits. Tsai tou vounou, lemon balm, bay leaf, and St. John's wort were most commonly used.

INTRODUCING THE HEALING PROPERTIES OF HERBAL TEAS

Herbal teas provide drinkers with a range of healthy benefits. Teas have long been regarded as a critical component of good health among Eastern cultures. More recently, Western researchers have invested time and energy in researching the benefits of various types of teas, including those of the herbal varieties.

First and foremost, most herbal teas do not contain caffeine, unlike any other tea. This property makes them ideal for providing calming effects. In fact, many different types of herbal teas are used to help with anxiety, stress, and insomnia, which would not be possible if they contained caffeine in any amount.

One significant benefit of many herbal teas is the antioxidants, vitamins, and minerals they provide drinkers. Depending on the type of herbal tea you drink, you can support your immune system with vitamins and minerals like folate, carotene, potassium, calcium, and magnesium. Many herbs have antioxidant properties, making them a great supplement to protect your body from damaging oxidation.

Some herbs can be used to make teas that promote better digestive health. These benefits range from aiding in morning sickness and nausea to constipation and diarrhea. Additionally, you can use some herbs to aid in managing chronic heartburn.

Herbal teas are a common source of stress and anxiety relief. Research indicates that several types of herbs can contribute to this effect. Studies have indicated a reduction in cortisol levels following the consumption of herbal tea, which indicates a related decrease in stress (Manaker, 2023).

Certain herbs can be selected to boost your immunity. These teas are beneficial during cold and flu season or just for generalized improved wellness. Depending on the herb you choose, this immunity-boosting benefit may be combined with other healing benefits to help you reduce the duration of sicknesses like the cold and flu that have no cure.

It's important to note that not every tea will provide all these benefits. The results you get boil down to the specific herbs you select. Each herb is unique in the healing properties it offers. I'll explain and detail many herbs as we continue our journey together.

WHERE TO FIND QUALITY AND AFFORDABLE INGREDIENTS

When choosing your herbs, finding the highest quality possible is essential to get the best benefits. In addition, you'll need to decide if you want to make your herbal teas with fresh or dried herbs. Both have their benefits, but it's important to know their differences.

Fresh herbs can vary in quality based on several factors, including how they were harvested, cared for, and handled during transport. Because of this, it can be quite a challenge to determine which are of the highest quality. When shopping for fresh herbs, you'll need to watch for vibrant colors that indicate the herbs are healthy and still at the peak of freshness. Any indication of browning could mean the herbs are aging. Additionally, you'll want those that appear to be freshly cut. The leaves should be intact, and you should not see any signs of decay or wilting. Finally, the highest quality fresh herbs will have a delectable aroma, whereas those of lower quality will have little to no aroma.

Dried herbs can be a bit more challenging than fresh herbs when finding the best quality. This is due to the effects of the drying process. Unfortunately, as herbs dry, they can lose some of their aroma and flavor. As you select your dried herbs, be mindful of any discoloration or deterioration of the packaging. It's also important to ensure the herbs are free from contamination such as dust. Any impurities indicate poor storage practices in place, making the herbs a much lower quality than you want. When you smell the herbs, you should not have any hint of mold or mustiness. Either will indicate a problem with the drying process in which some of the moisture was not removed from the herbs before packaging. Finally, high-quality dried herbs will have a much more intense aroma than lower-quality dried herbs. Additionally, their texture will be more pronounced.

When making herbal teas, it's up to you to decide which option is better for you. If you use fresh herbs, you must steep them to prevent loss of flavor. Boiling is not an option for this type of tea. You'll simply need to crush the leaves a bit before placing them into your teapot to steep. If you don't have access to fresh herbs or it's more convenient to keep dried herbs on hand, you can still receive the same benefits from your herbal tea.

You can easily dry fresh herbs at home if you prefer to keep dried herbs on hand for your teas. With several options to complete the process, you'll have all the herbs you need in no time. Two of the most commonly used methods are air-drying and oven-drying.

Air-drying has long been the popular method of drying herbs, especially in ancient apothecaries. To dry your herbs with this process, take a bundle of whole herbs that is no more than an inch in diameter and tie it together. In a dry space, hang your bundles upside down to dry. It's a best practice to label your herbs because once they dry, they have a striking resemblance to one another. Additionally, use a rubber band to tie the herbs together. The stems will shrink throughout the drying process, but the rubber band will securely hold them in place, preventing separation and falling. Once you are sure all the moisture has been removed from the herbs, take them down, crumble the dried leaves into a storage container, and store them in a cool spot out of direct sunlight for the best results.

Alternatively, you can air-dry herbs by plucking all the leaves from the fresh plant and placing them flat on a rack or sheet. However, with this method, you'll need to ensure the herbs are in a room without significant airflow, or there's a chance they'll blow away. You must ensure the room where you dry your herbs is dust-free, or you risk contaminating the batch.

The process takes roughly one week to complete with either method of air-drying. To test the dryness of your herbs, do a crumble test with a couple of leaves. They are ready to be stored if they easily break apart and feel completely dry.

The process is much quicker if you'd like to dry your herbs using an oven. When you select your herbs, remove any damaged or sickly parts. You'll need to wash the herbs, but ensure you're not overwashing so you do not add excess water. Note that if you do not use pesticides when growing your herbs, you may not need to wash them unless they are extremely dirty. If you buy herbs from the store, always rinse them. When using an oven, you must take care with the drying process because you can use too much heat. Your herbs will typically dry at a temperature of 222 °F (100 °C).

To get started, remove the stalks and place the herbs on a cookie sheet that's roughly an inch deep. Arrange the herbs so that you are maximizing the space used. There should be no more than one layer deep of herbs anywhere on the sheet. As you are heating the herbs, leave the oven door ajar. This will ensure excess heat can escape the oven, and any moisture released from the herbs will escape into the kitchen instead of remaining in the oven, preventing dehydration. Let the herbs sit in the heated oven for 20 minutes, flip them, and let them sit for another 10 minutes. You may need to repeat this process for two to four hours until the ideal consistency is achieved. Once the herbs are dry, cool them completely inside the oven.

When you source your herbs, choosing the best quality is essential. This ensures that you get maximum results from your herbal teas. Lower-quality herbs don't have the same potency and may be contaminated with chemicals. Sourcing certified organic herbs is ideal because you have the reassurance that your herbal teas are made with quality ingredients not grown with pesticides or herbicides.

To get the highest quality, it's best to shop locally. These herbs will be more potent than those shipped in from other locations. Additionally, sourcing locally is significantly more sustainable. Whether you want to buy from local markets or go wildcrafting to ethically pick your own from the wilderness, you can find premium options that haven't been damaged by transit.

If you don't have access to local markets or aren't comfortable harvesting in the wild, you can always buy from reputable online retailers. Researching and finding those with an excellent reputation for providing customers with the best products is essential. Some of the most reliable online retailers include:

- Monterey Bay Herb Co.
- Mountain Rose Herbs
- Starwest Botanicals
- Bulk Herb Store
- Frontier Co-op

One of the best ways to source high-quality herbs is to grow them yourself. You'll have complete control over the process, allowing you to keep your herbal tea preparations completely organic. You can also ensure they are always picked at their peak, which provides better potency, flavor, and benefits. When you grow your own plants, you'll need to select the varieties that grow best in your climate. Additionally, as you select your seedlings from a nursery, ensure you choose high-quality plants that show no signs of pests or diseases, as these can ruin your entire garden.

Another factor to consider when selecting your herbs is finding them at affordable prices. The most cost-effective way to obtain a steady supply of high-quality herbs is to grow them yourself. You'll need to make an initial investment in your garden, but once your plants start to grow, you can sustainably harvest them to continue providing fresh herbs throughout the growing season. If your garden is indoors, you may even enjoy year-round access to fresh herbs.

The second-best option is to utilize your local farmer's markets, bulk food stores, community gardens, and herbalists. All these local resources are more affordable because they generally don't ship their products in from far-off locations, effectively reducing their overhead costs and allowing them to offer reduced prices. These sources are also more inclined to offer the best quality products, ensuring you get the biggest bang for your buck.

Finally, you can turn to trusted online bulk herb retailers for excellent savings. You'll just need to remember that these herbs may not be as ideal as those you can purchase locally due to the handling required when shipping. However, many excellent retailers offer great products. These retailers include:

- Bulk Apothecary
- Bulk Herb Store
- The Spiceworks
- Spice Jungle

Remember, before choosing any online retailer, do your homework and ensure they have a solid reputation for only offering the highest quality products. Otherwise, it won't matter how much you save if you're getting the bottom of the barrel regarding quality.

TIPS FOR BREWING THE PERFECT TEA

While you can buy any number of premade herbal teas at your local grocery store, the problem is they're often full of artificial flavorings and lack the traits that make a legitimate herbal tea. To avoid these problems, the best option is to formulate your own herbal blends. It may seem as easy as throwing some herbs in a pot of hot water, but there's a bit more to create the ideal structure of an herbal tea.

The ideal herbal tea structure provides a range of flavors. To start, you'll need flowering notes. Calendula, dandelion, violet, and wild rose flowers often provide these. When making your tea, you'll want it to be one part flowering herb.

Next up is your placeholder flavor. This flavor ties all the components of your herbal tea together. Additionally, if you brew an iced tea, the flavor will remain stronger after the ice melts into the beverage. Common choices are dried raspberry leaves or dried nettles. Your tea will require two parts of this herb.

You'll also want to add a fruity component. This is a naturally sweet element. Many herbal tea drinkers use hibiscus flowers or dried rosehips for this part. Add one part of this component to your herbal tea mixture.

Finally, you'll want to add a cooling element. Mint, neem, and borage are commonly used as tea-cooling herbs. You'll finish up your recipe with one part of this herb.

Once you've decided on the herbs you will use to create your herbal tea, you must mix them. You can place them in a jar with a tight-fitting lid and gently shake the jar to thoroughly mix the herbs. This prevents damaging the herbs and ensures you get some of each in your brew.

There are two methods of preparing an herbal tea: infusions or decoctions. You can use a teapot, French press, infuser, or stainless steel pot to prepare an infusion. Place the desired amount of herbs in your container of choice and pour boiling water over the top of them. Place a cover on the container and steep for 20 minutes. Before drinking, strain the tea and discard the herbs. Alternatively, you can use a tea ball to hold the herbs during steeping. This makes it easier to remove them when the tea is ready.

When preparing a decoction, you'll make it on the stove in a stainless steel pot. This method is generally used for the harder parts of the herbs, including the bark and roots. Generally, you would not use this method to prepare herbal tea with leaves, as it can ruin the flavor. Place your herbs in the pot, add water, and bring the mixture to a boil. Once the water is boiling, reduce the heat and simmer for 20 to 30 minutes while covered. When the time is up, strain the herbs and enjoy your tea. Depending on how well your herbs hold up during the simmering process, you may be able to use them again for another decoction. Refrigerate them between uses.

As you can see, herbal teas have a rich history. From ancient times, they have been used to heal various ailments and offer an excellent alternative to coffee and regular tea. From sourcing high-quality herbs to blending potent herbal teas, you now have all the information you need on the fundamentals of these beneficial drinks. In the next chapter, we'll focus on taking a holistic approach to wellness.

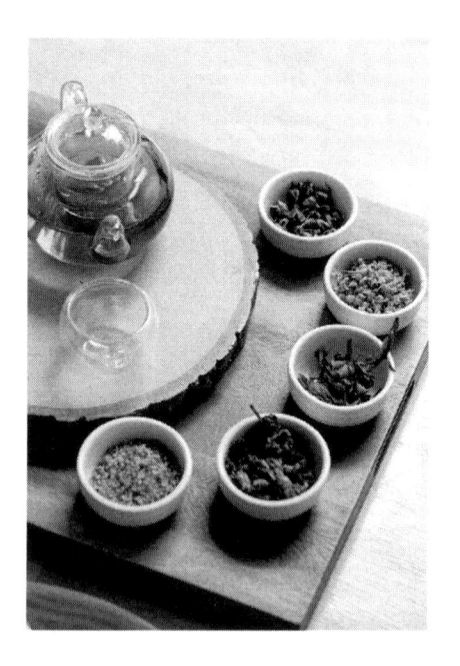

2

BALANCE FOR A HOLISTIC APPROACH TO WELLNESS

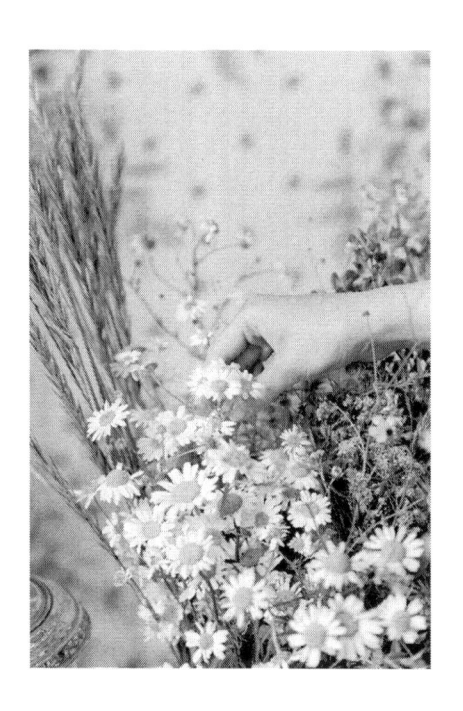

> *Enjoy life sip by sip, not gulp by gulp.*
>
> — THE MINISTER OF LEAVES

Drinking tea provides more than just a solution to slake your thirst; it can be an invaluable tool to achieve a state of calm and an overall holistic approach to health and wellness, providing a sense of calm and healing during trying times.

One such trying time was the COVID-19 pandemic. Many individuals found themselves seeking solace for stress and anxiety during this bleak period of isolation. While tea isn't a cure-all for all your problems in life, it can provide a much-needed respite.

For one woman, 2020 was a year of enforced solitude that left her needing comfort. The lack of social interaction was a heavy weight that needed to be lifted. To find that solace, she drank tea each day, using her own specific ritual. While it didn't fix everything, it provided solace and structure that helped ease her loneliness (Kelly, 2020).

With this in mind, we'll use this chapter to consider the importance of a holistic wellness approach, including tea rituals and meditation. You can reap more benefits from your tea-drinking experience by incorporating rituals and mindfulness.

THE IMPORTANCE OF TAKING A HOLISTIC APPROACH TO WELLNESS

"Holistic wellness" has become quite the buzz phrase in recent years, but it's not a new concept. Despite its popularity, defining it can be a bit confusing. For those who have consistently taken a conventional approach to health and wellness, it's generally understood that mainstream medical practitioners look at the individual symptoms and ailments, focusing on treating them. This can leave the door open to missing so many aspects of the individual's overall wellness.

On the other hand, holistic wellness views the entire person. When you take a holistic approach to health and healing, you consider all aspects, including your physical, mental, and spiritual health. It is implicitly understood that considering the person as a whole is essential to the overall pursuit of health and spiritual wellness. Instead of simply considering the specific ailment or symptoms, a holistic approach views all aspects of your life to find where you need healing. Ultimately, holistic wellness seeks to get to the heart of health and wellness problems, not just eliminate the symptoms. This is often done by finding a place of balance, healing, and positive energy.

Holistic wellness is essential to helping you reach a state of optimal health. Once you're there, it will also help you maintain it. Optimal health is unique to everyone, so what you strive for may not be the same as your friends and family. However, with a holistic approach to your health and wellness, you focus on your entire well-being, which generally leads to long-term wellness. No matter who you are or how you experience optimal health, it generally features having good physical, emotional, and spiritual balance, having vitality and energy that allow you to do the things you enjoy, and feeling great mentally and emotionally.

Taking a holistic approach is important when caring for your health and wellness. It allows for a deeper understanding of the underlying conditions and true causes of any mental or physical ailments you are experiencing. Instead of just focusing on the symptoms of your problems, this approach will allow you to get down to the root cause. It is important to note that your symptoms will still be addressed, but you'll take things further to discover what has led to these problems.

There is no single way to achieve holistic wellness. You can perform a variety of routines and activities that will promote your overall health and wellness with a holistic approach. While herbal teas are a great addition to your daily routine for moving toward a holistic lifestyle, you should also focus on several other aspects of your health and wellness, including:

- eating a healthy diet
- getting regular exercise
- staying hydrated
- aiming for the recommended amount of sleep nightly
- practicing self-care to promote mental and emotional wellness
- nurturing your relationships to fulfill your social wellness needs
- seeking medical advice for ailments and conditions

Eating a healthy diet is essential because food is your fuel throughout the day. It's what keeps you going and gives you energy. When you choose unhealthy foods, it can take a toll on your health and wellness. Eating the right foods supplies the nutrients you need for optimal physical health and wellness.

In addition to a good, balanced diet, you need to move your body daily. Exercise helps you physically and stimulates the flow of neurotransmitters like endorphins that boost your mood. It can reduce the effects of stress and help with symptoms of depression as more neurotransmitters are released. Combining exercise and a healthy diet can also lead to weight management that can ensure you reach and maintain an ideal weight for your needs.

With all the popular drinks available today, many overlook drinking pure, unadulterated water. Our bodies need to be properly hydrated to function normally. Water keeps our brains at peak performance and ensures our organs operate optimally.

Many of us have busy lifestyles that don't leave much time for much-needed relaxation. However, getting the recommended amount of sleep each night is critical to your health and wellness. Once in a while, you can get by with missing a couple of those precious hours of sleep, but the more days you miss, the more the effects will compound. Sleep is essential for all aspects of your health, including the physical, mental, and emotional aspects.

Self-care is another important aspect of holistic wellness. When you take the time out of your busy schedule to tend to your own needs, you'll develop better mental and physical wellness.

When you improve your physical health, you'll have greater mental and emotional health results. Eating a whole diet, exercising, and getting enough sleep all work together to improve your physical well-being, which, in turn, stimulates a positive response in your mental and emotional well-being. Additionally, caring for your emotional and mental needs can improve physical health as you reduce stress and anxiety.

Your relationships also play an important role in holistic wellness. Social health gives you a sense of belonging and inspires you. Your interpretation of yourself often comes from how those in your life see you. This includes how well your self-esteem develops. You want to seek out relationships that bring fulfillment to your life. Nurturing these relationships will bring positivity to your life.

You should also have a medical professional you can turn to when you have ailments and conditions that need more treatment than your holistic lifestyle can provide. Holistic wellness will provide the foundation you need to live a more fulfilling and healthy life, but there are times when you may need the guidance of a medical professional.

AN INTRODUCTION TO TEA-DRINKING RITUALS

While a holistic approach is an exceptional way to take on your wellness journey, the same approach toward tea drinking is also highly beneficial. One of the best ways to do this is by participating in tea-drinking rituals. You likely have some of your own well-established rituals and understand that these practices give your life structure and meaning. When you engage in rituals, you connect with your deeply hidden inner self, create stability, and bring a sense of order to a life often lived with an abundance of chaos.

Tea rituals are essentially a ceremonial method of tea preparation and consumption. Like any other healing and comforting ritual, stopping to consume a cup of tea can provide significant relief to those participating. A tea ritual provides a break from the hustle and bustle of daily life, a much-needed moment of peace, and a deeper human connection that we often lack when interacting with others.

Tea ceremonies have a lot of cultural significance and can be found in many countries worldwide. Many ceremonies and rituals exist in different countries and revolve around various types of teas.

In China, the ceremony is called Cha-Dao, which translates into the "way of the tea." Dao is a prevalent philosophy in China that promotes a life in harmony with the nature surrounding you. Many interpretations of Dao exist, but the prevailing themes include simplicity, balance, patience, the realization that all things will change, and the idea of "going with the flow." Cha-Dao presents the unique opportunity to interpret and fully comprehend the Dao by drinking tea. Other ceremonies common in China include the wedding tea ceremony, Wu-Wo tea ceremony, and perennial tea ceremony.

Japanese traditions use the Chanoyu tea ceremony. While tea drinking was introduced to the country during the 8th century, green tea is a common morning beverage today. It is also enjoyed periodically throughout the day. As in China, the

Japanese ceremony Chanoyu is another translation of "the way of the tea." It is based around matcha. However, this ceremony is more about preparing the tea and making ceremonial gestures than drinking the green tea. Each detail is designed to please the guests and induce Zen meditation by expressing simplicity and creating elegance. Matcha ceremonies are typically conducted in a traditional-style tearoom and offer a bonding experience that includes respect, honor, appreciation, hospitality, and mindfulness.

The primary tea of India is chai, which is a blend of black tea, herbs, and spices that are boiled in milk and water. Because of its popularity, there are chaiwalas, or those who prepare and serve chai, nearly anywhere you go in India. Its origins date back to 5,000 to 9,000 years ago. While chai is enjoyed throughout the day, it is a common practice to drink it at approximately 4 p.m. while enjoying an afternoon snack. Despite the country's evolution, it is still common for many individuals to migrate toward the small roadside chai stands to watch a small family operation brew this tea steeped in tradition.

In Morocco, tea drinking didn't become a mainstream practice until the mid-19th century. The primary tea is Tuareg tea, a green tea blended with mint leaves and sugar. Other herbs are frequently added, including absinthium. When a Moroccan family has a guest at their home, it is a tradition and expectation that they will offer the guest tea. This practice demonstrates hospitality and friendship. During the traditional tea ceremony, the tea is prepared before the guest; however, with modernization, many have moved to prepare the beverage in the kitchen separate from the guest.

Despite these countries' rituals pairing with specific teas, it's important to note that any tea can be enjoyed at any time in a relaxing manner. You can take the time out of your day and enjoy your own tea ritual with your chosen tea.

Tea rituals are a source of great comfort, especially during troubling times. The story of one woman's childhood sums this up quite well. Jasmin was raised in a home deeply rooted in tradition with her Persian family. Her father adored tea well beyond its ritualistic use for offering hospitality to guests. The family would make tea first thing in the morning and refresh it throughout the day. If guests came to visit, they would be offered tea until they accepted. From preparation to serving to drinking, the entire process was ritualistic. Now that Jasmin has become an adult and no longer lives in Iran, she still practices the ritual of drinking tea throughout her day. It provides great relief from anxiety and stress and can help induce sleep for her. Additionally, taking a break to enjoy the teatime ritual offers a respite from the monotony and pressures of the day. The rituals she learned as a child are something she still practices today as an adult in the United States (Tahmaseb-McConatha, 2022).

While many tea-drinking rituals seem complex, when you create your own, you don't have to make it challenging to perform. Instead, try to minimize all the fuss, keeping things simple. Teatime should be a deeply personal experience. You can consider adding a sweet treat, which is common among tea rituals, but you don't have to. Additionally, you are not required to break out the fine china.

You do not have to set a specific time to enjoy tea. Teatime can be any time of day. Consider what works best for you. The average teatime is approximately 30 minutes long, so you'll need to factor that into the equation when determining when you'll drink your soothing tea blend.

There's something special about tea. It's not like coffee or soda that you can drink while working. Instead, it's a drink you'll want to savor, which means taking a step away from work, phone, and other distractions. Teatime is time you set aside for yourself and can be considered self-care. Because of this, you'll need to set boundaries to ensure you can enjoy your cup in peace.

You can make your tea ritual even more special when you include loved ones. This might be surprising, but kids can also enjoy a good cup of tea. When you come together and take a break from the hustle and bustle of life, you can experience a bonding moment that you won't get from other activities.

Making your own tea ritual is highly beneficial because you can create the perfect environment to generate clarity, calmness, and stillness. You can create the same beneficial effects as meditation when you create the ideal tea ritual to serve your needs. To do this, you'll need to take several necessary steps.

First, you need to set the stage. When you decide to hold a tea ritual, you must clear physical space and set aside the required time. It's important to remember that steeping requirements cannot be shortened. You must follow them to the letter to ensure your tea turns out correctly. In addition to steeping time, you'll need time to thoroughly enjoy the tea without distraction. If you have 15 minutes to spare, that can be enough for your ritual. Because it is a ritual, you'll want to establish the same items each time you perform it. These items can include the same tea set, a specific type of tea, and the same location.

As you perform each action, make them gently. The physical act of drinking is only a minute part of the tea ritual. It starts with opening your mind and concludes with a thankful appreciation for your generated positivity. Additionally, you can also set the tone for the ceremony. This step can include reading a poem, praying, or simply sitting in silence.

During your tea ritual, you may be interested in doing another activity. Ensure it is relaxing and doesn't detract from the ritual itself. Consider meditation, coloring, or enjoying a tasty snack.

When you're ready to bring your ritual to a close, take a moment to appreciate the time you've spent. Before heading back to work or another hectic task, be grateful for the peace you've just enjoyed.

INCORPORATING MEDITATION AND MINDFULNESS WITH TEA DRINKING

When you incorporate meditation and mindfulness practices into your tea drinking, you take another step toward holistic wellness. Mindfulness is doing something with purpose and intent, fully aware of the present moment. Taking time to be fully present in the moment and aware of yourself and your surroundings leads to a better holistic approach to your overall health and wellness. Meditation is an approach that helps keep you focused to achieve a state of mindfulness. When you meditate, you focus on clearing your mind, which can help alleviate stress and anxiety. As you reach a state of mindfulness, you also cultivate heightened sensory awareness.

Practicing mindfulness offers several significant benefits. One of the primary benefits is the reduction in depression. Mindfulness can reduce the symptoms associated with depression and help prevent them from returning in the future. Similarly, it can also aid in your ability to regulate your emotions. If you have difficulties controlling how you respond to different situations, mindfulness can help give you the control you need to reign in your emotions as needed. Mindfulness also reduces stress and anxiety by helping you address thoughts, behaviors, and feelings that contribute to them.

Mindfulness also presents individuals with a better ability to manage illness. The practice often gives those with chronic illnesses the help they need to handle their symptoms. It won't present a cure for those symptoms, but it can allow the individual to better manage them.

Mindfulness will improve your mental and physical health and overall well-being. You can enjoy significant benefits from reducing blood pressure to improving sleep by including mindfulness in your daily routines. You'll be able to deal with challenges that surface, improve your self-esteem, and form deeper connections with those in your close-knit circle.

Meditation offers quite a few similar benefits to mindfulness. You can decrease depression, stress, and anxiety. Additionally, meditation is an excellent tool to improve emotional health and well-being. Through breathing techniques and centering your mind, you can help control your emotions.

It's also an excellent tool for increasing your self-awareness. The more you practice meditation, the more you will get to know yourself and how you relate to the world surrounding you. Because meditation requires you to continually refocus your mind, it helps boost your attention span. Meditation can also strengthen the immune system, reduce hypertension and the risk of heart disease, and increase your ability to avoid job burnout.

Mindfulness and meditation can be implemented in your tea rituals. From brewing to drinking, they can have a powerful impact on your tea session's effects. To incorporate these practices into your tea routine, start with the brewing process. Focus on moving your tea leaves from the packaging to your cup. From there, watch as your tea leaves unfurl in the hot water. With each movement you make, consider what you are doing and how you are moving. During this process, there are so many details you can take in that it can be overwhelming, so don't focus on everything at once. Be present in the moment, consider your actions, and focus on the task at hand, not your surroundings or distractions.

When it's time to drink your tea, you can continue being mindful and meditating. Think about the flavors of the tea as they hit your tongue. Consider what's happening to your body as you drink. You don't need to define anything you're tasting. Instead, enjoy the moment and take it all in. Again, limit your distractions to just you and your tea. Live in the moment, enjoying the experience as it happens. As you take each sip, savor the flavor and feeling. It's also important to embrace the stillness of the activity.

A holistic approach to your health and wellness is essential to reach optimal health. Incorporating tea drinking with holistic elements can be an excellent way to enhance your approach. The act of drinking tea is more than just about consuming a drink—it's a total mind and body experience that should be enjoyed, from brewing to drinking. In the next chapter, we will consider the different safety precautions you should take to minimize the risk when consuming herbal teas.

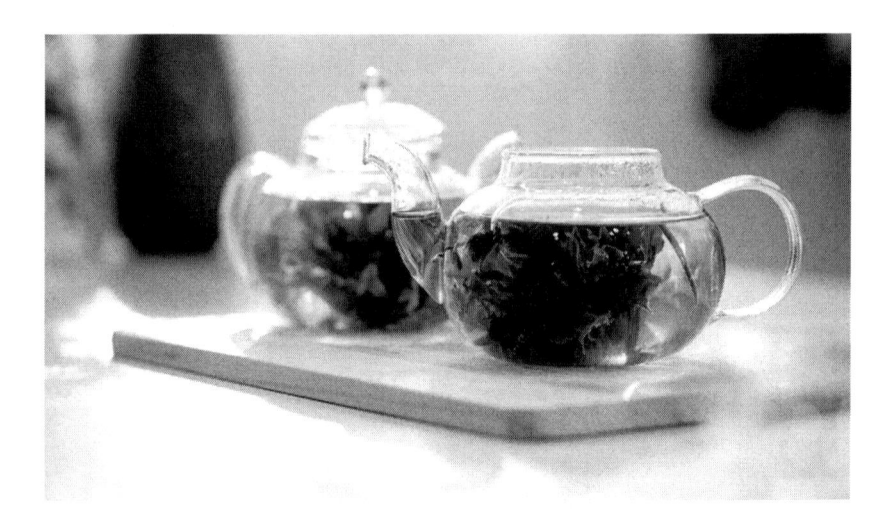

3

A GUIDE TO SIPPING SAFELY AND MINIMIZING RISK

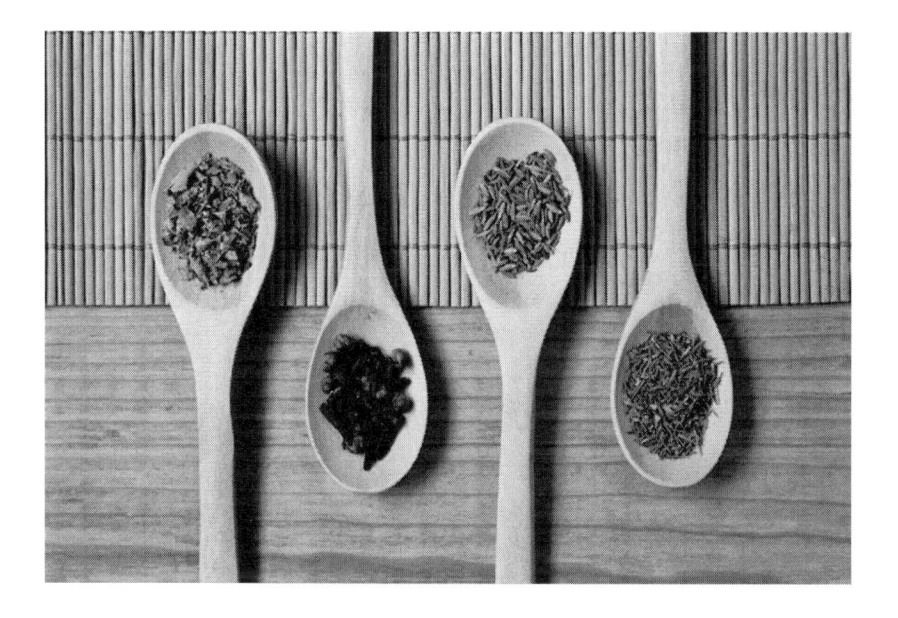

" *Tea is the elixir of life.*

— EISAI, KISSA YOJOKI

Herbal tea offers significant benefits to those who enjoy drinking it. However, it's not without its risks. Knowing what these risks are and how to avoid them is key to ensuring you can carefully sip your tea and enjoy all the positive effects it brings.

In this chapter, we'll focus on how you can safely drink your herbal tea. We'll start by considering the potential risks. We'll also explore how to prepare your tea and when to consult with your physician.

POTENTIAL RISKS OF HERBAL TEAS TO CONSIDER

While drinking tea seems innocent enough, you will need to consider some potential risks. For instance, caffeine should only be consumed in moderation. It is perhaps the most apparent reason that drinking too much tea could make you feel ill. The caffeine content of tea varies significantly based on the type you select. However, herbal teas are generally caffeine free.

When you ingest too much caffeine, you'll generally experience any or all of the following symptoms:

- headache
- dizziness
- racing heart
- anxiety
- stress
- restlessness

- poor sleep
- heartburn
- complications in pregnancy
- caffeine dependence

Tea generally comes with its caffeine content on the packaging. Any tea derived from the actual tea plant will contain caffeine. This includes black tea and green tea. Because herbal teas aren't actually made from the tea plant, they generally have no caffeine-containing substances.

Another considerable risk with tea drinking is the presence of toxins in commercially available products. Unfortunately, several major tea brands contain toxic chemicals but have no disclosure on the packaging. If the toxin levels in your tea are high and you consume a large quantity of the tea, you are at risk for severe complications. Some of the toxins commonly found in commercially produced teas include:

- DDE: a derivative of the banned substance DDT
- heptachlor epoxide: a version of the U.S.-banned heptachlor that was once used to kill termites until it was found to cause cancer
- permethrin: a chemical that can harm the endocrine system and has been linked to cancer
- acetamiprid: a chemical used to kill bees
- fluoride: while naturally occurring and not technically toxic, too much will cause harm

Drinking too much tea can impose many significant side effects on your body. To begin with, it can decrease your body's ability to absorb iron, which will lead to a deficiency. The reason this happens is because tea contains a high percentage of the compounds called tannins. These compounds bind to iron in certain types of food, making it unavailable for absorption within your gastrointestinal tract. Iron deficiency is one of the world's most common deficiencies, and if you struggle with it, drinking tea could worsen it. The level of tannins varies according to the type of tea you're drinking.

Because of the caffeine content in traditional teas, consuming a large amount of tea can result in increased restlessness, anxiety, and stress. In general, black teas tend to contain the most caffeine, with green and white teas having a lower caffeine content. However, the longer you steep your tea, the greater the caffeine concentration will be. When you notice signs of being jittery, it's likely time to cut back on your tea intake or switch to non-caffeinated herbal blends.

Depending on when you consume your tea and how sensitive you are to caffeine, you could also affect your ability to get a good night's sleep. For some, consuming a cup of tea within two hours of bedtime is enough caffeine to disrupt that night's rest.

Too much tea can also lead to digestive issues, such as nausea and general abdominal discomfort. The tannin content can irritate digestive tissues, resulting in these symptoms. For some, as little as one cup can produce complications, while others can drink more than five cups and never develop a single problem.

Another digestive problem tea can inflame is heartburn, especially in those with acid reflux problems. Caffeine releases the sphincter that separates the esophagus and stomach. This allows stomach acid to easily flow into the esophagus. Additionally, caffeine may be responsible for boosting the production of stomach acid.

Pregnant women are often advised by their physicians to avoid consuming too much caffeine. Drinking too much tea is no exception. When consumed in excess, caffeine can lead to miscarriages or low birth weights. The jury is still out on what exactly is a safe amount of caffeine during pregnancy.

While infrequent use of caffeine is related to a decrease in headache pain, the opposite is true for chronic consumption. When you drink too much tea, the caffeine can actually cause headaches. Additionally, while rare, excessive caffeine consumption can lead to dizziness. So, if you're drinking a lot of tea and start to feel lightheaded, it could be the cause.

The more tea you drink, the more caffeine you consume. In turn, this can lead to caffeine dependence. Caffeine dependence can lead to an abundance of other problems, including headaches, increased heart rate, fatigue, and irritability when you experience any amount of withdrawal from it.

It's not very common, but it is possible to be allergic to tea. The symptoms of a tea allergy include hives, tingling in the mouth, swelling in the mouth or face, and anaphylaxis. If this happens, you could be allergic to the caffeine content, tannins, or theanine.

A GUIDE TO RESPONSIBLE HERBAL TEA CONSUMPTION

When you stop to consider how much herbal tea you should consume each day, certain factors will play a major part in determining this. For instance, your current overall health plays a significant role in the amount of any herb you should consume. The other factors include your gender, age, and weight. However, the average adult can typically consume two to three cups of herbal tea daily with no unwanted side effects. This is just a general rule and should be reconsidered in cases where the drinker is pregnant, breastfeeding, or taking certain medications.

Preparing an herbal tea comes with some typical requirements as well. In general, when brewing your tea, you should use only 1 to 2 teaspoons of dried herbs or 2 to 4 teaspoons of fresh herbs with each cup of water. You should soak your chosen herbs in the hot water for approximately five to ten minutes before straining and serving. Again, this is just a general rule. The amount of herbs you use can vary based on your specific needs, the herb you are using, and how strong you want your tea to be.

In addition to these guidelines, you'll also want to ensure you know all your allergies. Herbs are like any other food or supplement you might consume in that they can cause an allergic reaction. Because of this, it's essential to know if you're allergic to the herbs you intend to use before you brew your first cup of herbal tea.

Some commonly used herbs also have negative interactions with certain medications. One specific example is St. John's wort. While it offers a host of benefits, including aiding in the management of moderate depression, it can cause antidepressants to not work correctly. It's best to consult with your physician if you are on any medications to ensure your herbal teas will not impact your treatments in any way.

As with any food, herbs have the potential to be contaminated with pesticides and heavy metals. It's important to protect yourself by purchasing yours only from trusted sources. Spending a bit extra on certified organic products can give you peace of mind knowing that your herbs were grown without chemicals. Look for that special seal on the packaging.

WHEN IN DOUBT, TALK TO A DOCTOR

While herbal tea can provide a lot of positive support for your health and well-being, it is not a cure-all. When you're in doubt about anything, it's time to see your doctor. Mental health is often challenging to discuss, but it's something that needs to be brought up if you're experiencing any problems. These conditions are often mild, but in extreme cases, they can cause a significant risk to your life and safety. Not talking about them can put you at risk of placing yourself in a dangerous situation. Hiding your symptoms will not make them go away. Instead, take that step, no matter how scary, and discuss your concerns with a professional.

In addition to seeking help for mental health concerns, you should also bring up any physical health issues. Your doctor will help you by working through the various symptoms to come up with the proper diagnosis. They'll find the ideal treatment option. This is also the perfect time to discuss whether your herbal tea is compatible with your therapy.

Herbal tea can provide many benefits, but you must not rely on these teas alone. Some ailments require the aid of a physician or other medical practitioner. Whether you have mental or physical health concerns, it's best not to try to self-treat all the time. A doctor is your best bet for getting the treatment you need and knowing if your herbal tea is the right choice for you.

If you're ever on the fence about your choice of herbal tea, don't be afraid to ask your doctor. They'll know whether your tea interacts with any of your medications or conditions. They'll also be able to tell you whether you're consuming too much. Even if they are not holistic medical practitioners, conventional medical doctors will still have essential knowledge related to the use of herbal teas.

While herbal teas can provide many healthy benefits to drinkers, there are several risks you need to pay attention to. It's important to consult with your physician if you're on any medications to ensure your herbal tea will not adversely react with them. In the next chapter, we'll focus on the benefits of using herbal tea for stress and anxiety.

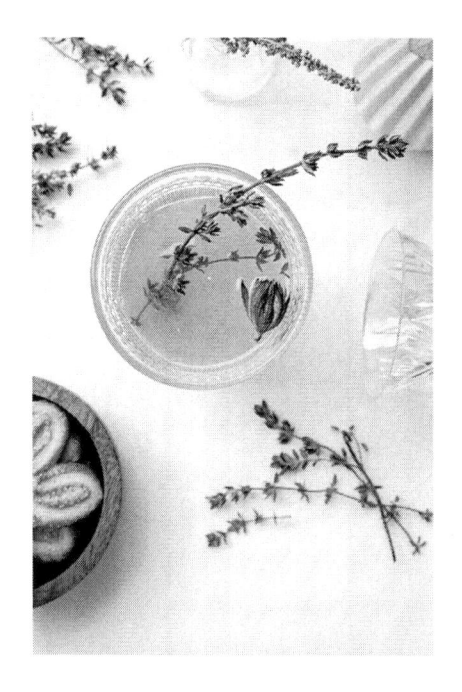

HERBAL TEAS SIMPLIFIED | 51

4

BECOME CHAMOMILE CALM WITH STRESS-RELIEVING TEAS

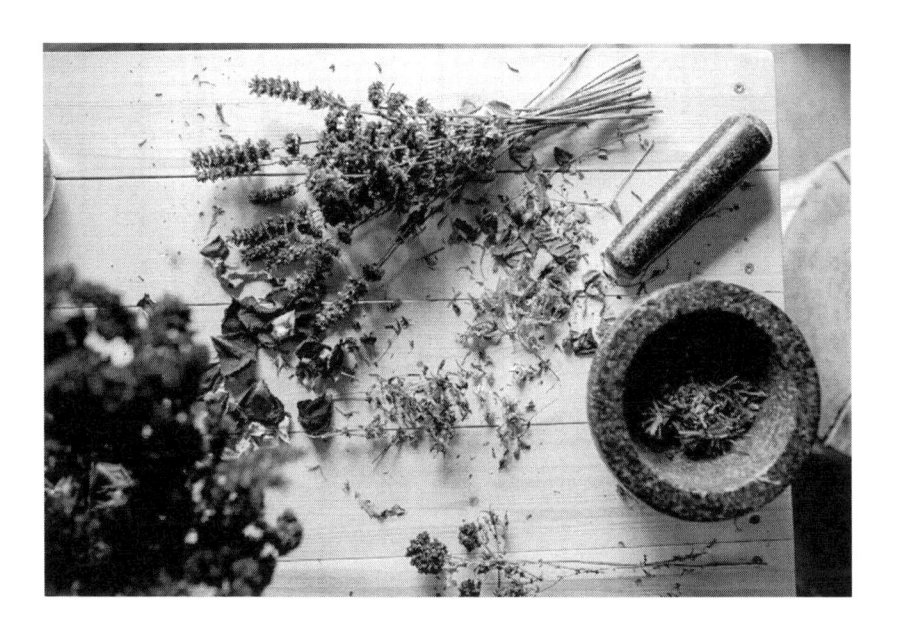

The tea session is modeled after the silence of retreat; a time to enjoy life far removed from daily existence.

— SEN JOO

There's no doubt that today's world is full of stress and anxiety. It can be challenging to make it through one day without something popping up that stimulates either of these responses.

Over the centuries, many have relied upon herbal teas to help cope with symptoms of stress and anxiety. Because of their proven history of efficacy, those herbs are still used today.

We'll start this chapter with an exploration of what stress and anxiety are. Understanding these two responses is essential to finding the best way to manage them.

UNDERSTANDING STRESS AND ANXIETY

We talk about stress and how it can negatively affect your health and well-being, but what exactly is it? Essentially, stress can be identified as a change that strains you physically, emotionally, or psychologically. While this may sound alarming at first, stress is a natural response to any situation you perceive as potentially dangerous.

Sudden stress causes your brain to flood your body with various chemicals and hormones that, in turn, cause increased heart rate and greater blood flow to critical muscles and organs. It triggers a sense of heightened awareness, allowing you to focus on the immediate needs of the situation.

Everyone experiences stress in their lives. Your response will determine how it affects your overall well-being. Depending on the specific circumstances, the best solution may be changing your situation or how you respond to the situation.

There are three types of stress you should be familiar with. They include chronic stress, acute stress, and episodic acute stress. Chronic stress feels like it's never-ending and like something you will never escape from. This type of stress can come from childhood trauma and other traumatic experiences. Acute stress is the short-term stress we undergo daily, which can be positive or negative. One specific type of acute stress is episodic acute stress. It differs in that it runs wild and never seems to quit, creating a perpetual state of distress.

Many different aspects of life can cause stress, including parental responsibilities, workload, financial problems, interpersonal relationships, and general inconveniences that can occur daily. Some examples of acute and chronic stressors include:

- caring for a loved one with a chronic illness
- living with your own chronic illness
- being in an unhappy or abusive relationship
- enduring a prolonged divorce battle
- living at or below poverty conditions
- experiencing little to no work-life balance
- working at a job you cannot stand
- being deployed or having a loved one deployed
- surviving a life-threatening incident or illness

Regardless of what has caused your stress, there are some universal symptoms. You may experience some or all of them, depending on the amount of stress you're feeling. Between feeling overwhelmed, fearful, or irritable, you may also experience any of the following symptoms:

- chronic pain
- sleep problems
- appetite changes
- inability to concentrate or make decisions
- decreased sex drive
- fatigue
- digestive problems

While the stress response is normal, it can have severe impacts on your health and well-being, especially when it becomes chronic. You may find that as you experience stress, it's harder to manage the daily hassles you face, your interpersonal relationships are negatively impacted, and your health faces detrimental impacts.

Stress over certain situations, like money, your living situation, or a relationship, can cause physical illness and other health concerns. As your brain experiences increased stress, your body will respond in kind.

If you have severe acute stress, the situation can cause significant health problems, including heart attacks and sudden death. However, it should be noted that these outcomes are more commonly associated with individuals who already have heart disease.

Some forms of stress can induce mild anxiety and frustration, while prolonged bouts of stress can lead to burnout, depression, and anxiety disorders. Chronic stress can lead to an overactive autonomic nervous system, which causes bodily damage.

One way to help stem the flow of stress is to initiate the relaxation response. This method involves a combination of approaches, including deep abdominal breathing, visualization techniques, yoga, repetitive prayer, tai chi, and focusing on soothing words. Research has been conducted on using the relaxation response to reduce chronic stress in those with hypertension. The results demonstrated that those who effectively used the relaxation response could reduce their hypertension significantly enough to eliminate at least one of their blood pressure medications (*Understanding the Stress Response*, 2020).

Another way you can reduce the stress response is by drinking tea with mindfulness, meditation, and rituals. When you practice mindfulness, you are fully present in the moment. While you're experiencing everything, you can recognize stressors and allow them to move past you without affecting you the way they would under normal circumstances. As you meditate, your focus is on the present, while you clear your thoughts and open your mind. These tea-drinking rituals help organize a world full of chaos into something more manageable, allowing you to handle your stress.

Anxiety is a state of negative expectation experienced both physically and mentally. On the mental side of things, anxiety is typified by heightened arousal and apprehension that present themselves as a distressing state of worry. In the physical sense, you'll experience the overall activation of multiple systems within your body that help you respond to real or imagined danger. These associated feelings of dread and the accompanying physical sensations are designed to create feelings of discomfort. The purpose of anxiety is to capture your attention and make you aware of the current situation. With that awareness, you will be stimulated to take action to protect all that is important to you. Experiencing occasional anxiety can be natural and even beneficially productive.

Everyday anxiety is classified as worry over common things in your life, such as bills, getting a job, or even a breakup. It can relate to an embarrassing situation that causes you to feel uncomfortable or awkward. Additionally, this type of anxiety can be associated with jitters before a big test, stage fright, or fear before another big event. Everyday anxiety can also occur when you fear something dangerous, whether it's a person, place, or object. You may also experience anxiety immediately following a traumatic event, causing you to have trouble sleeping or sadness related to the incident.

Severe anxiety differs significantly from everyday anxiety. It is classified as severe, chronic, and unsubstantiated worry that interferes with your daily life, causing significant distress. It can lead to you completely avoiding social situations out of the fear of being judged or humiliated. You may experience panic attacks that seem to come from nowhere and live in fear of another one popping up. Severe anxiety can also cause a powerful and irrational fear of harmless objects, places, and people. You may also experience recurring nightmares, flashbacks, or other psychological problems related to a traumatic incident that happened several months or more before.

The signs of anxiety are more than just whirls of worry throughout your mind. You'll also experience a gamut of physical symptoms, including jumpiness, trembling, ringing in the ears, increased breathing rate, and a pounding heart.

Anxiety is caused by being human and having the ability to envision what the future may hold. It is unique in that real-world events can trigger it, or it can be entirely generated through thoughts relating to a threat, whether real or imagined. In this way, anxiety has the potential to be caused by external events or internal thought patterns.

Many experience what is known as the cycle of anxiety. When an anxiety-triggering event occurs, the individual may feel as if they have no control or experience a significant amount of fear. Because of this, they avoid coping with the situation to escape from any intense emotions. This avoidance helps to perpetuate the cycle, further triggering themselves. Instead of relieving their anxiety, they cause their symptoms to increase, including having more anxiety, panic, and worry.

The cycle of anxiety is typically experienced in four stages:

- Stage one: You have anxious feelings and want to deal with them.
- Stage two: You make a solid attempt to avoid the situation.
- Stage three: You have a temporary sense of relief from the act of avoidance.

- Stage four: You return to a heightened state of anxiety.

Your fight-or-flight response kicks in automatically when you're in stage one. In the second stage, you're likely to experience bodily reactions geared toward self-protection. Based on what happens in stage two, you feel some respite from your anxiety in stage three, but once stage four arrives, you're likely to feel drained on all fronts, mentally, emotionally, and physically.

Taking the time out of your day to mindfully sip a cup of tea can help ease your anxiety. You can soothe your worry by getting to the heart of it using mindfulness techniques, meditation, and tea rituals. The ritual action of tea drinking can provide you with a sense of control where you once felt lacking. In addition, bringing mindfulness into your life allows you more awareness of your feelings and their sources.

A GUIDE TO NATURE'S CALMING HERBS

Many different herbs present stress and anxiety-relieving properties, making them excellent candidates for your stress-relief tea. When you need to find that calming, soothing source of relaxation, these are the ideal herbs.

Used since the 16th century, lemon balm is well-known for its sedative effects. This herb is a member of the mint family and offers several benefits, including stress and anxiety reduction, sleep disruption abatement, and digestive problem reduction. Studies conducted on lemon balm products indicate they have the potential to positively impact mood and stress (Caplan, 2021).

Green tea isn't an herb but is often used in herbal tea blends. However, it offers several mood-boosting effects, including protection against oxidative stress and improved mood memory and response times. Research has found that those who consistently drink green tea tend to have lower stress levels than those who do not, as it can reduce anxiety and stress levels when regularly used (Coelho, 2022).

Chamomile has long been used to reduce symptoms of anxiety and stress. This herb offers tea drinkers sedative and relaxing properties. It is highly beneficial in the reduction of symptoms of generalized anxiety disorder. However, it cannot prevent future symptoms from recurring. One of the key ingredients in chamomile is the flavonoid apigenin. In studies conducted on mice, apigenin effectively reverses stress, repairs memory, and provides an antidepressant effect. Additionally, chamomile has demonstrated excellent results as a natural sleep aid (Lamoreaux, 2022).

The first use of lavender dates back to medieval times when it was used for its calming effects. It's beneficial as a sleep aid. Enjoying lavender tea at bedtime has long been a solution for getting the best night's sleep. Lavender calms the nervous system, easing problems with disturbed sleep, anxiety, and restlessness. Additionally, it may boost the benefit of reducing depression in older adults, according to studies. The primary benefit of lavender is its ability to bring about calm without inducing a sedative effect (Lamoreaux, 2022).

Peppermint is an all-natural way to knock out your stress. Simply smelling its powerful aroma can bring about a reduction in the pain and anxiety associated with catheterization. It's especially beneficial to those hospitalized for heart attack and childbirth, as it can reduce the associated symptoms of stress and anxiety.

Another relaxing herb is gotu kola. It is often used in Asian cultures as a form of traditional medicine or in a tonic. The primary use has been to treat fatigue, depression, and anxiety. If you're struggling with insomnia and other sleep problems, drinking a tea made from gotu kola may be just what you need.

For those with a racing, busy mind, passionflower is just what the doctor ordered. It provides an overall calming sensation that leads to the mind slowing down, allowing for a restful night's sleep. It's an excellent herb to be used for the reduction of anxiety.

Hailing from the world of Ayurvedic medicine, ashwagandha aids in treating anxiety. Studies have demonstrated its efficacy in reducing stress and anxiety (Coelho, 2022). Ashwagandha is an adaptogenic herb, which makes it ideal for stress reduction.

Tulsi, or holy basil, has been regularly used for physical and mental health benefits. It is known for aiding in the reduction of the symptoms of general anxiety disorder. It also has pain-relieving properties, which can reduce stress and anxiety.

St. John's wort is one of the most used herbs for the treatment and management of mild to moderate depression. It is also one of the most thoroughly studied options. While the focus has been primarily on depression, it is an excellent option for helping to manage anxiety. It may positively affect stress and stress-inducing hormones, lowering the user's symptoms. However, care must be taken with this herb to ensure there are no interactions with current medications.

You've likely heard of catnip for stimulating cats into playtime. However, when used in humans, it provides the complete opposite effect. Catnip tea is one of the most soothing drinks, as it relieves the symptoms of anxiety. Additionally, drinkers are likely to experience a good night's sleep due to the calming effects.

ANXIETY AND STRESS-RELIEF TEA RECIPES

While there are many great options for herbs to bring about anxiety and stress relief, you're likely interested in learning what recipes make the most of them. I have a ton of great recipes to share with you that I think will benefit you most in reducing your anxiety and stress symptoms.

Soothing Sweet Tea Blend

This tea blend is a bit minty with sweet undertones. Its flavors are less on the herbal side and more on the floral. The mint provides that essential relaxation you're looking for, while the other flavors keep the tea slightly sweet and tart.

Ingredients:

- 1 tsp mint

- 1 tsp dried rosehip
- 1 tsp hibiscus flower (Katja, 2017)

Directions:

1. Combine all ingredients in your teacup.
2. Boil 8 ounces of water.
3. Pour the water over your herbal blend.
4. Steep for 5–10 minutes.
5. Strain the tea and enjoy.

Calming Stress-Relief Tea Recipe

Lavender and chamomile are excellent choices for stress relief, and this tea uses both. Lemon balm adds an extra kick to the blend and is a nice sleep aid.

Ingredients:

- 1 tsp lavender
- 1 tsp chamomile
- 1 tsp lemon balm (Katja, 2017)

Directions:

1. Combine the three ingredients in your tea cup or tea ball.
2. Boil 8 ounces of water.
3. Pour the water over the herbs.
4. Steep for 5–10 minutes.

5. Strain the tea before enjoying.

Autumn Tea Blend

This tea is the best choice if you're looking for a refreshing blend that suits the cooler autumn weather. It combines lemon balm and peppermint for soothing results when anxiety and stress peak.

Ingredients:

- 1 tsp stinging nettle
- 1 tsp dried rosehip
- 1 tsp lemon balm
- 1 tsp peppermint
- ½ cinnamon stick (Katja, 2017)

Directions:

1. Blend the first four ingredients in your teacup.
2. Boil 8 ounces of water.
3. Pour the water over the herbs.
4. Steep between 5–10 minutes.
5. Strain the tea, add the cinnamon stick, and enjoy.

Calming Tea Recipe

This calming tea recipe is ideal for stress management. It offers a holistic approach to any self-care routine and can enhance overall well-being. Note that when measuring this recipe, you can use any measurement for the parts if you are consistent, depending on the amount of tea you want to make.

Ingredients:

- 2 parts lemon balm leaf
- 1 part chamomile flowers
- 1 part linden bract and flower
- 1 part rose petal
- ½ part spearmint leaf

Directions:

1. Thoroughly blend the herbs in a bowl and store them in a sealed glass container until ready to use.
2. Place 1–2 tablespoons of the herbal tea blend in a teacup.
3. Pour 1 cup of boiling water over the blend, cover it, and steep it for 10–15 minutes.
4. Strain the tea and enjoy.

You can drink this tea 3–4 times daily for stress relief and relaxation (Karen, 2020).

Lavender Orange Tea

This tea is highly versatile and can be served hot or cold. Additionally, you can substitute other citrus fruits for the orange slices, depending on the flavor profile you'd like to enjoy.

Ingredients:

- 2 tsp dried lavender flowers
- 1–2 fresh slices of orange
- 1 tsp honey, optional
- 8 oz water

Directions:

1. Combine the lavender flowers with water in a small saucepan.
2. Simmer over medium-high heat, stirring constantly.
3. Remove from heat and strain.
4. Serve with orange slices and honey.

This recipe makes one serving (Paleohacks, 2016).

Lemon and Ginger Calming Tonic

Whether you need to calm your stress and anxiety levels or open your sinuses, this tonic does it all. The added magnesium boosts stress reduction, ensuring you have a great day.

Ingredients:

- 1 tsp grated fresh ginger root
- 1 tbsp lemon-flavored magnesium
- 1 sliced fresh lemon
- raw honey

Directions:

1. Combine ginger, honey, and boiling water.
2. Add lemon slices to each mug you have prepared.
3. Serve the tea warm (*Lemon and Ginger Calming Tonic*, n.d.).

Chamomile Tea Latte

This soothing, caffeine-free recipe uses a French press to froth the milk. It's simple to make and ready in just eight minutes.

Ingredients:

- 2 cups milk
- 1 cinnamon stick
- 5 crushed cloves
- 2 tbsp loose-leaf chamomile tea
- 2 tsp vanilla extract
- ground cinnamon

Directions:

1. Combine milk, cinnamon stick, cloves, and chamomile tea leaves in a saucepan.
2. Simmer on low heat.
3. Strain the resulting latte into a French press and add the vanilla extract.
4. Close the lid and pump until the latte doubles in size.
5. Pour the latte into mugs, garnishing with ground cinnamon (Choe, 2018).

Lemon Balm Tea

This lemon balm tea is perfect if you're interested in a super easy tea recipe for relieving stress and anxiety. It requires two ingredients: herbs and water.

Ingredients:

- 3 tbsp dried lemon balm
- 3 cups boiled water

Directions:

1. Place lemon balm in a large mason jar or teapot.
2. Pour boiling water over the herbs.
3. Steep for 10 minutes.
4. Strain and enjoy immediately (Susannah, 2022).

Lemon Mint Iced Tea

For this recipe, you'll need to choose a quality base tea. This can be chamomile tea or another soothing herbal blend that goes well with mint.

Ingredients:

- 1 sliced lemon
- 1 sliced lime
- 8 fresh mint leaves
- ice cubes
- 3 cups of your chosen herbal tea, chilled

Directions:

1. Place the lemon and lime slices in a jar with the mint.
2. Fill the jar with ice cubes and chilled herbal tea.
3. Refrigerate for 4–6 hours (Rick, 2023).

Lavender Iced Tea

This tea combines lavender with Earl Grey tea. It offers a soothing remedy for stress and anxiety; however, due to traditional tea being included, it's best not to drink this option before bed.

Ingredients:

- 8 cups boiling water

- 6–8 bags of Earl Grey tea (if using loose-leaf tea, use 1½–2 tbsp)
- 1–1½ tsp dried lavender flowers
- ¾ cup simple syrup
- pinch of baking soda
- pinch of sea salt

Directions:

1. Combine boiling water, tea, and lavender in a large heatproof bowl. If you're using loose-leaf tea, use a tea ball to contain the lavender and tea leaves.
2. Steep for 10 minutes
3. While steeping, add simple syrup, baking soda, and salt. Stir well to combine.
4. Adjust the tea to your taste, adding more syrup for sweetness and water to make it less intense.
5. After steeping, strain the tea and allow it to cool to room temperature.
6. Chill in the refrigerator before serving (Asha, 2020).

Jack Frost Tea

Jack Frost tea combines soothing peppermint with spearmint to bring about a reduction in stress and anxiety. You'll enjoy its naturally sweet flavor as you sit back and relax.

Ingredients:

- ¼ cup dried peppermint leaves

- ¼ cup dried spearmint leaves

Directions:

1. Combine the herbs in a glass jar and shake well to combine.
2. Use 1 teaspoon of herbal blend per 8 ounces of water.
3. Add the desired amount of tea and water to a teapot.
4. Steep for 5–10 minutes (Stanley, 2012).

Lemon Ginger Tea

If you're on the hunt for a tasty, soothing drink, try this lemon ginger tea recipe. With its refreshing citrus and ginger combination, you'll be coming back for more in no time.

Ingredients:

- 4 cups boiling water
- 2 in. ginger root, sliced thin
- 1 sliced lemon

Directions:

1. Boil water and remove from heat.
2. Add ginger and lemon while the water is still hot.
3. Steep for 20 minutes.
4. Serve cold or hot (Johnson, 2019).

Homemade Dried Fruit and Herb Tea

This interesting blend offers several soothing properties for your overall health. With its decadent combination of dried fruits and herbs, you'll be relaxing in no time.

Ingredients:

- zest of 2 oranges, finely chopped
- zest of 2 lemons, finely chopped
- 3 in. ginger, finely chopped
- ½ small fennel bulb, finely chopped
- 1 cup packed fresh mint leaves
- 1 cup dried cranberries

Directions:

1. Preheat your oven to 250 °F (121 °C).
2. Combine orange zest, lemon zest, ginger, and fennel on a parchment paper-lined baking sheet.
3. Place mint on an additional parchment paper-lined baking sheet.
4. Bake both sheets, rotating and stirring periodically. Continue until both mixtures are dried out.
5. Allow both baking sheets to cool fully.
6. Crumble the dried mint into a medium mixing bowl.
7. Add the ginger mixture and cranberries. Toss to combine.
8. Steep 2 tablespoons of the blend for 3–5 minutes in 1 cup of boiling water.

9. Strain the tea before serving (*Homemade Dried Fruit and Herb Tea*, n.d.).

Ginger Mint Green Iced Tea

While this tea is a nice alternative to coffee, it's still made with green tea, which means you shouldn't drink it close to bedtime. It's best to enjoy this blend in moderation.

Ingredients:

- 3 in. unpeeled ginger, thinly sliced
- 6 cups water
- 6 green tea bags
- 1½ cups loosely packed fresh mint leaves
- additional mint leaves for serving
- ⅓–½ cup honey
- 1–2 tbsp freshly squeezed lemon juice
- ice

Directions:

1. Add the ginger and water to a saucepan and bring to a boil over high heat.
2. Immediately remove the pan from the heat once the water boils.
3. Add the tea bags and mint.
4. Steep covered for 15 minutes.
5. Strain the tea into a large pitcher.
6. Refrigerate to chill for at least one hour.

7. Before serving, add ⅓ cup of honey and 1 tablespoon of lemon juice. Add more of either to taste.
8. Serve in tall glasses with ice using more mint as a garnish (Mollenkamp, 2015).

Relaxation Tea

Look no further than this relaxation tea when you need a solid blend for relaxation and stress relief. It takes advantage of the positive benefits of many excellent anxiety-reducing herbs.

Ingredients:

- 2 parts chamomile flowers
- 1 part passionflower
- 2 parts lemon balm
- 1 part oat straw
- 1 park skullcap
- 1 part ginger

Directions:

1. Combine all ingredients in an airtight container. Shake well to combine.
2. Use 1–2 tablespoons of your herbal blend with 8 ounces of hot water.
3. Strain before drinking (Villegas, 2022).

DIY Stress-Relief Tea

This stress-relief tea is a perfect blend of herbs chosen specifically for their ability to target the nervous system. By doing this, they aid in reducing and balancing stress levels. Each herb chosen has a holistic effect when supporting the body.

Ingredients:

- ½ tsp dried eleuthero root
- 1 tsp dried lemon balm
- 1 tsp dried chamomile
- ½ tsp dried lavender
- 2 tsp dried holy basil

Directions:

Combine all ingredients in a cup.

1. Pour hot water over the top and cover.
2. Infuse for 20 minutes.
3. Uncover and filter the tea.
4. Add any desired sweetener and enjoy (Lederle, 2019).

Passionflower, Lemongrass, and Chamomile Tea

Passionflower is known for its powerful anti-anxiety properties. This tea takes advantage of those properties and further boosts them with the effects of lemongrass and chamomile.

Ingredients:

- 1 tbsp dried passionflower petals
- 1 tsp dried lemongrass leaves
- 1 tsp dried chamomile
- 1 cup boiling water

Directions:

1. Combine the herbs.
2. Pour the boiling water over the herbs.
3. Steep for 10 minutes.
4. Strain and add your sweetener of choice (Camila, 2022).

Decaf Herbal Stress-Relief Tea

While this tea takes a bit of effort to make, it's well worth it in the end. You'll benefit from a great immune boost and reduced stress.

Ingredients:

- 2 cinnamon sticks
- 10 black peppercorns
- 1 in. fresh ginger, sliced
- 1 tsp cardamom
- ½ tsp whole cloves
- ½ tsp fennel seeds
- 2 cups milk
- 1 tbsp honey

- 2 bags decaf black tea

Directions:

1. Create a makeshift tea bag with gauze and string. Place the cinnamon sticks, peppercorns, ginger, cardamom, cloves, and fennel seeds inside this tea bag.
2. In a large pot, add the milk and honey.
3. Add the decaf black tea and your makeshift tea bag to the milk.
4. Bring the milk to a low boil and steep the mixture for at least 10 minutes.
5. Remove all tea bags before serving (Power of Positivity, 2021).

Chamomile, Lavender, and Rose Tea

These three herbs complement each other well with their delicate flavors. In addition, they each offer exceptional stress-relieving benefits.

Ingredients:

- 1 part dried chamomile
- 1 part dried lavender
- 1 part dried rose petals

Directions:

1. Place 1 teaspoon of your herbal blend into a pot with 1 cup of water and the lid on.
2. Bring the mixture to a boil and immediately turn the heat off.
3. Steep for 15 minutes.
4. Strain the tea into your cup.
5. Add any milk or sweetener you want and enjoy (Loewe, 2022).

Lemon Balm and Chamomile Tea

Lemon balm and chamomile pair well for their anxiety and stress-reducing properties. This tea is very easy to make and will have you sipping on a soothing blend in no time.

Ingredients:

- 1 part dried lemon balm
- 1 part dried chamomile

Directions:

1. Combine 1 teaspoon of your herbal blend with 1 cup of water in a small pot with the lid on.
2. Bring the water to a boil and immediately turn the heat off.
3. Allow the mixture to steep for 15 minutes.
4. Strain the tea into your preferred container.

5. Add milk or sweetener to taste (Loewe, 2022).

INTERACTIVE ELEMENT

While many practice a full tea ceremony to take advantage of the meditative benefits of the process, you don't have to be so formal. Drinking a cup of tea at some point in your day is enough to get started. To practice a tea meditation, there are a few key steps you'll need to take:

1. Select your tea.
2. Carefully and meaningfully choose your cup.
3. Observe the water as it boils.
4. Watch as the tea transitions from its leaf form into the brew you drink.
5. Mindfully savor each sip, focusing on the tea's flavor and feel as you drink.
6. Enjoy the process, focusing on the physical act of drinking the tea and pushing off thoughts of rushing through the act.
7. Finish your tea meditation with thoughts and actions filled with gratitude for the experience.

As you take the time to embrace your tea drinking from start to finish, you'll be more mindful about your stress and anxiety. It's a great way to bring your concerns to the forefront of your mind and release them. Tea meditation is a great way to exhibit mindfulness in your daily routines.

Herbal teas have many exceptional benefits when it comes to easing the symptoms of stress and anxiety. With so many options available, you can experiment until you find the ideal herbal blend that suits your needs. In the next chapter, we'll change our focus slightly to dial into using herbal teas for sleep aids.

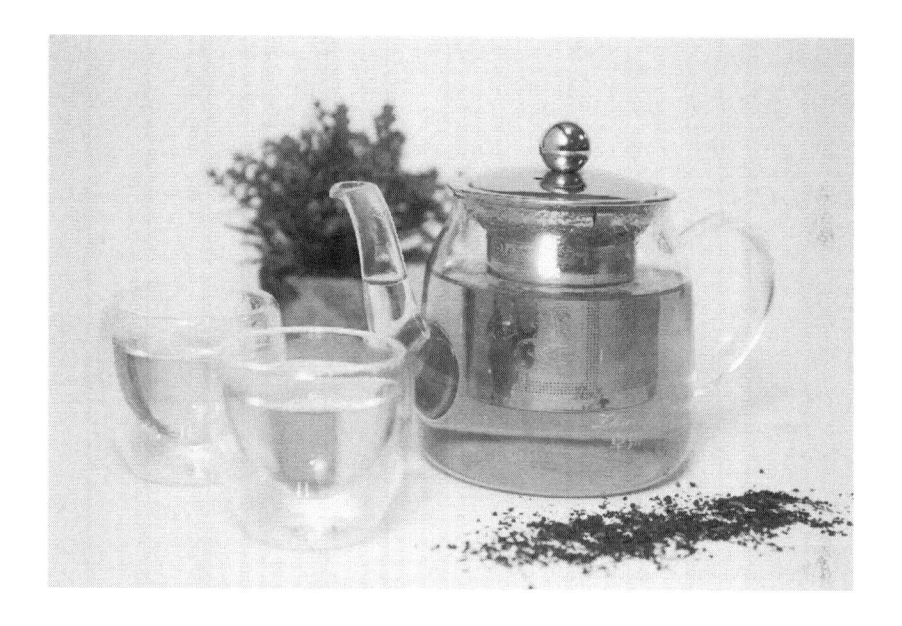

Filling the Teapot for the Whole Community

"Herbs are the natural healers of the world."

— UNKNOWN

I don't claim to know the exact chain of events that brought you on this journey of discovering the healing powers of herbal teas, but I'd hazard a guess that you were sick of spending vast amounts of money on over-the-counter remedies that left you with side effects more irritating than the ailments you started with.

The pharmaceutical industry has made sure we rely on it, often at the expense of our own health, and we've become further removed from the natural treatments we could have been using (to much greater effect) all along.

Everyone has the power to make use of herbal teas to improve their health and overall quality of life. The problem is that not everyone knows how to do so, and with the food and medicine industries doing everything they can to line their pockets, it's hard to see a clear path.

I wrote this book to light that path and help more people discover the huge potential and transformative powers of herbal teas. Now that you've come this far along the road, I'd like to ask for your help in reaching more people. The good news is it's incredibly easy: all you have to do is leave a short review.

By leaving a review of this book on Amazon, you'll help other people who are looking for a natural way to tackle both mental and physical health issues to find all the guidance they need.

Your words have enormous power, and this one small act will light the way for new readers, helping more people discover the wonders of herbal teas for good health.

Thank you so much for your support. There's a lot of noise out there, but together, we can light the way to a more natural and effective way of taking good care of our health.

Scan the QR code to leave a review!

5

EXPERIENCE VALERIAN DREAMS WITH SLEEP-INDUCING TEAS

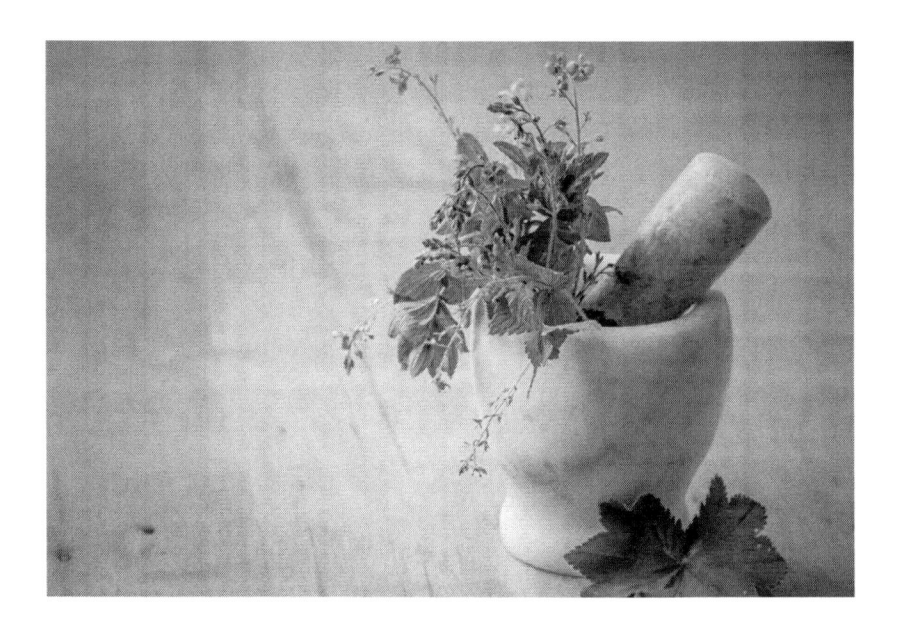

> *Tea time is a chance to slow down, pull back, and appreciate our surroundings.*
>
> — LETITIA BALDRIGE

Sleep doesn't always come easy for everyone. In fact, many suffer from sleep disorders or simply cannot get their brains to slow down when it's time for bed. Erica was one of those people until she did some research on sleep-inducing herbal teas. From chamomile to lavender to valerian, she found several options that helped calm her stress, ease her mind, and soothe her into a calm state to get a restful night's sleep.

It wasn't just about the soothing herbs in her tea for Erica. It also extended to the ritual of making and drinking it. To avoid the complications associated with sleeping medications, she added this ritual to her nightly routine. Since that first cup of herbal tea, she's been able to get a full, restful night's sleep.

In this chapter, we'll explore why sleep is so important and the different herbs that can provide a calming effect to help you find your way to dreamland more easily. Let's start with the science behind this essential bodily function.

THE SCIENCE OF SLEEP

You may not think about what happens when you sleep, but it's a lot more than just closing your eyes and dreaming. The sleep cycle has four stages, each with a different effect on your brain. The first three stages are part of non-rapid eye movement (NREM) sleep. The fourth is the only one that is considered rapid eye movement (REM) sleep.

The first stage of sleep is essentially a transition period. It lasts for approximately one to five minutes and covers the move from dozing to stage two. In the second stage, your brain and body continue to slow their activity. This stage can take anywhere from 10 to 60 minutes to complete. You're more easily awakened during these first two stages, as you have not entered a deeper sleep.

In stage three, your muscles and body relax more. Your brain waves are markedly different from those in a waking stage. This deep sleep phase is essential for bodily recuperation, effective thinking, and reliable memory. Stage three typically lasts for 20 to 40 minutes.

Stage four is the only REM stage of the sleep cycle. During this stage, your brain activity experiences a significant boost, while most of your body goes into temporary paralysis except for the respiratory muscles and eyes. REM sleep is essential for brain support, enabling memory and learning. It is more common in the later parts of the night and can occur for 10 to 60 minutes at a time.

Different things happen to your body as you progress through the sleep cycle. During the three NREM stages, breathing slows. It ultimately reaches its lowest rate during the deepest sleep of stage three. However, once you enter REM sleep in stage four, your breathing will increase and potentially become irregular.

Similarly, during the first three stages, you'll experience a reduction in your heart rate. It will reach its lowest rate during stage three but again pick up the pace in stage four. In fact, it will reach a rate similar to what your heart rate is during regular waking hours.

Throughout NREM sleep, your muscle tone changes as your body enters a complete state of relaxation. The total amount of energy your body expends also significantly decreases. As I previously mentioned, your body will enter a state of paralysis called atonia during REM sleep. This is to prevent flailing of your limbs during the dream state. Your eyes will stay very active behind your lids, and your breathing will remain active.

Sleep is essential in maintaining various hormone levels in your body. As you progress through the stages, the levels of these hormones will fluctuate, and poor sleep can lead to complications. Sleep-related hormones include cortisol, growth hormone, leptin, ghrelin, and melatonin.

While you may dream during any stage of the sleep cycle, there is a marked difference between the dreams you will experience in NREM sleep and those in REM sleep. Because REM sleep dreams are more vivid, they also tend to be more fanciful, bizarre, and immersive.

The body controls sleep with the help of your circadian rhythms and sleep drive. Circadian rhythms can be considered a type of biological clock that exists deep within the brain. This clock recognizes light cues throughout the day. When the lights are off and daylight ends, the brain produces melatonin. Then, when the lights come on and the sun comes up, the melatonin production stops.

On the other hand, sleep drive is your body's response to the need for sleep. As you progress throughout your day, this need intensifies. Once this need reaches its peak, you will ultimately succumb to it and sleep. The need for sleep is not like hunger.

For example, no matter how intense the feelings are, your body cannot force you to eat when you're hungry. However, if you're exhausted, it can shut down everything and put you to sleep, no matter where you are.

The National Institutes of Health (NIH) recommends the average adult should get between seven and nine hours of sleep nightly. Sleeping fewer than seven hours each night can lead to health complications that those who sleep seven hours or more do not face. Sleeping more than nine hours may not be harmful, especially for those recovering from sleep deprivation complications or an illness (*How Much Sleep Is Enough?* 2022).

Sleep is an essential biological function we all need to survive. Children use their time sleeping for physical and mental development. When adults get the right amount of sleep, they are better able to ward off certain negative health consequences ranging from cardiovascular problems to depression and anxiety. While having one bad night of sleep is generally something you can recover from, having multiple in a row can lead to any of these health problems. Because of this, planning your day to allow enough time for restful sleep and finding ways to manage sleeping problems is essential.

A GUIDE TO NATURE'S SLEEP AIDS

If you need the aid of a natural sleep-inducing herbal tea, you won't be disappointed with the variety of herbs you can use. These herbs all work to deliver good-quality sleep that will leave you well-rested the following morning.

Valerian root is a commonly used sleep aid. It's well-known for its ability to aid in overcoming insomnia, anxiety, and restlessness to help people get a good night's rest. It contains a compound called valerenic acid. This compound is responsible for inhibiting the breakdown of GABA, a neurotransmitter. In addition to improving sleep, valerian can help you fall asleep faster.

Because it has powerful relaxation properties, passionflower is another excellent sleep aid. It contains several nerve-relaxing flavonoids, which are responsible for aiding in getting better sleep. When passionflower tea is consumed in the evening, it leads to a better overall quality of sleep with improved feelings of refreshment the next day. Additionally, it can also reduce the likelihood of waking in the night.

Ashwagandha functions as an all-natural sedative, which means it can help you fall asleep faster and stay asleep. The herb contains triethylene glycol, which can relieve sleep anxiety. This can also help improve the regulation of your sleep cycles.

Another excellent option for rest and relaxation at bedtime is skullcap. It provides a source of relaxation for the mind and body, ensuring you can wind down adequately before falling asleep.

Hops have been studied and found to induce better-quality sleep in participants. In addition, other studies have demonstrated its efficacy in supporting those with insomnia, allowing them to fall asleep more easily and stay asleep (Powers, 2022).

You need chamomile if you're looking for an herb with a long history of successful use in producing relaxing effects. Modern-day studies have also confirmed the efficacy of this herb. It's a great solution for easing insomnia. It contains nerve-relaxing flavonoids, which effectively make it a tranquilizing substance (Osmun, 2020).

Blue vervain has a history of traditional use as a sleep aid in many cultures. As demonstrated in an animal study, it contains two phytochemical compounds, hastatoside and verbenalin, which likely improve sleep quality. Additionally, blue vervain has demonstrated an ability to reduce sleep latency and increase REM and NREM sleep stages (Powers, 2022).

Kava kava can improve overall sleep quality while reducing sleep-related anxiety. It is a safe and effective natural supplement for aiding in anxiety-related sleep problems.

Magnolia bark is great for helping people fall asleep faster while improving the overall quality of their sleep. Additionally, it reduces cortisol levels in the body, which reduces feelings of anxiety and stress. It's important to note that if you try this herb as a sleep aid, you should not use it during the day unless you intend to go right to sleep. It's that effective.

Jujube contains several important compounds that aid in sleep. The presence of saponins can help improve sleep time and induce an overall sleep-inducing effect. The flavonoid spinosin can reduce sleep latency while improving the night's sleep duration.

You've likely heard of lavender used as a sleep-inducing tea, as it is the most commonly used herb for that purpose. Lavender can help improve your wakefulness the following morning by decreasing grogginess. Additionally, it's beneficial in aiding in managing mild insomnia while improving overall sleep quality.

Holy basil works to promote sleep by reducing stress and anxiety. It contains adaptogens that your body naturally uses to combat stress. Adaptogens work to balance your mental state while preventing stressors from impeding your ability to sleep. Holy basil is also a good choice for relieving aches and pains that can keep you up at night.

St. John's wort contains tryptophan, which helps boost serotonin production. Because of this, it is commonly used to combat depression and its symptoms. This property aids in improving sleep patterns.

Mint teas are also remarkable for their pleasant flavors while aiding in sleep. Peppermint tea offers natural muscle-relaxing properties that can ease the built-up tension throughout your body, setting you up for success with a good night's sleep.

Lemon balm offers the same benefits as mint teas, likely because it comes from the same family. However, lemon balm offers a pleasing alternative if you're not interested in a minty-flavored tea.

California poppy aids in getting better sleep by reducing your aches and pains. This herb is a great option if you're looking for a natural alternative to pain medications. It also promotes relaxation to help you ease into sleep more quickly.

Ginseng is most often associated with improving one's cognitive abilities. However, it can also slow your thinking processes, allowing you to sleep soundly through the fog of mental fatigue.

SLEEP-ENHANCING TEA RECIPES

In this section, I will share the recipes I have found to be the most enjoyable and helpful for getting a good night's sleep. They're all easy to make and well worth the effort that goes into them.

Sweet Sleep Tea

Sometimes, you just need to relax and de-stress before hitting the hay. This tea recipe combines chamomile, lavender, and rose with a touch of honey to lull you into a peaceful sleep.

Ingredients:

- coconut or pasteurized raw milk
- ½ cup chamomile flowers
- ¼ cup dried orange peel
- ¼ cup lavender buds
- 2 tbsp rose petals
- raw honey

Directions:

1. Combine chamomile, lavender, rose, and orange and store in an airtight glass jar.
2. To brew, place 2 teaspoons of the herbal mixture into a cup.
3. Heat 8 ounces of water until boiling and pour it over the tea blend.
4. Steep for 3–5 minutes.
5. Strain the tea before serving.
6. Add milk and honey to taste (Jamie, 2014).

Cinnamon Sleep Tonic

When insomnia strikes, this tea blend can hit back hard. You'll be sleeping well in no time once you enjoy this flavorful brew.

Ingredients:

- 2 in. fresh ginger, cut into large pieces
- 1 tbsp allspice berries
- 10 cups filtered water
- ½ tsp peppercorns
- 3 cinnamon sticks
- 15 bay leaves
- 1 tbsp cloves

Directions:

1. Combine all ingredients in a saucepan and bring to a boil.
2. Reduce heat and steep for 2–3 hours before serving.

You can add cream, butter, honey, or coconut oil to the tea, but you can also drink it plain (*Herbal Tea Recipe for Sleep*, 2013).

The Ultimate Herbal Blend Tea

While you can buy a commercially produced herbal blend for your nightly routine, you don't have a lot of control over what goes into it. This ultimate herbal blend puts you back in the driver's seat when you prepare your homemade tea.

Ingredients:

- 1 oz dried lavender
- 1 oz dried chamomile
- 1 oz dried lemon balm
- 1 oz dried passionflower

Directions:

1. Combine all ingredients in an airtight container, preferably glass. Store out of direct sunlight.
2. When ready to make a cup of tea, add 1 cup of boiling water to 1 tablespoon of the tea blend and steep for 10–15 minutes.

3. Drink the tea while it's hot, inhaling the vapors with each sip (*Herbal Sleep Tea*, 2014).

Valerian Tea

Valerian tea is a great solution for insomnia as it works to encourage the brain cells to produce more GABA, which soothes the nerves and relieves anxiety.

Ingredients:

- 1 tsp valerian root

Directions:

1. Place the valerian root in a tea diffuser and into an empty container.
2. Boil 8 ounces of water.
3. Pour over the diffuser.
4. Steep while covered for 15 minutes.
5. Strain the tea into a cup and enjoy (Panchal, 2019).

Cuddle Time Tea

This tea recipe is ideal for total mind and body relaxation and stress reduction. It's a great option for aiding with anxiety and insomnia.

Ingredients:

- chamomile, rooibos tea
- peppermint leaves
- vanilla essence

Directions:

1. Combine all ingredients.
2. Use 1½ teaspoons of herbal mixture with a 16-ounce cup.
3. Add boiling water to the cup and steep for 3–5 minutes (Panchal, 2019).

Moonrise Herbal Tea

When you need a soothing herbal blend, consider this recipe. It combines chamomile's benefits with other sleep-inducing herbs, including lavender and skullcap.

Ingredients:

- 2 parts chamomile flowers
- ½ part lavender flowers
- ¼ part valerian root
- 1 part passionflower
- ¼ part hop flowers
- 2 parts lemon balm
- 2 parts skullcap

Directions:

1. Measure all ingredients into a mixing bowl.
2. Mix gently until well combined.
3. Store in an airtight container in a cool, dark location until ready to use.
4. Brew your desired amount of herbal blend in a single-serve cup and enjoy it before bed (Panchal, 2019).

Passionflower and Lavender Tea

The combination of passionflower and lavender makes for a soothing, calming blend. It also has a tasty, fruity flavor you'll love.

Ingredients:

- 1 part lavender blossoms
- 2 parts hibiscus flowers
- 2 parts passionflower
- 1 part chamomile
- 2 parts catnip

Directions:

1. Combine all ingredients in a container and mix well.
2. Place your desired amount of herbal blend into a cup.
3. Boil water and pour over the herbs.
4. Steep for 5–10 minutes.
5. Strain before enjoying (Dessinger, 2015).

Chamomile and Licorice Blend

This tea blend combines three calming herbs with the delicious flavor of licorice. Once you taste it, you'll be ready to incorporate it into your daily routine.

Ingredients:

- 1 part chamomile flowers
- 1 part lavender blossoms
- 1 part licorice root
- 1 part catnip

Directions:

1. Combine all ingredients in a bowl and stir well.
2. Add the desired amount of herbal blend to a cup.
3. Pour boiling water over the tea blend.
4. Steep for 5–10 minutes.
5. Strain before drinking (Dessinger, 2015).

Great Night's Sleep Tea

When you need to kick your nighttime routine into high gear to get the best sleep possible, try this tea made from a trifecta of sleep-inducing herbs.

Ingredients:

- 4½ cups water
- 1 tbsp dried lavender

- 3 tbsp dried chamomile
- 1 tbsp dried lemon balm

Directions:

1. Bring the water to a boil and reduce to a simmer.
2. Add the herbs to the water.
3. Cover and simmer on low for 15 minutes.
4. Strain and enjoy (Bryant Shrader, 2021).

Banana Peel Sleep Tea

Banana peel is a surprising source of magnesium and potassium, which can aid in getting a restful night's sleep. This tea uses this property and combines this beneficial ingredient with several herbs.

Ingredients:

- 2½ cups filtered water
- 2 banana peels
- 2 cinnamon sticks, 3 in. each
- 4 tsp loose-leaf chamomile tea
- 4 tsp loose-leaf lemon verbena tea
- 4 tsp loose-leaf lemon balm tea
- 1 tsp fennel seed

Directions:

1. Combine water, banana peels, and cinnamon sticks in a saucepan.
2. Bring the water to a boil and immediately turn the heat off.
3. Add chamomile, lemon verbena, lemon balm, and fennel seeds to the water.
4. Cover and steep for 10 or more minutes.
5. Strain into a mug to serve (Lucy, 2022).

Sleep Herbal Tea

While chamomile is one of the most popular sleep aid choices, not everyone enjoys it. This tea is the perfect alternative if you'd rather skip it.

Ingredients:

- 1 part passionflower
- 2 parts lemon balm
- 1 part lemongrass
- 1 part rose petals
- 1 part lavender
- 1 part valerian
- 1 part linden

Directions:

1. Combine all ingredients and place in an airtight container.
2. Combine boiling water and 1 tablespoon of the herbal tea.
3. Steep for 5–7 minutes while covered.
4. Strain and enjoy (Daniela, 2018).

Bedtime Tea

This tea is the perfect blend to enjoy about an hour before bed to soothe you into the right mindset to get a good night's sleep.

Ingredients:

- 1 tsp dried passionflower
- 1 tsp dried lemon balm
- 1 tsp dried chamomile
- 1 cup boiling water
- 1 tsp raw honey

Directions:

1. Combine the herbs and place them into a tea ball inside a mug.
2. Add boiling water and honey.
3. Steep until you reach your desired potency and flavor (Kelly, 2021).

Ginseng Tea

Ginseng tea is a uniquely refreshing beverage that provides all the necessary soothing properties to help you fall asleep quickly.

Ingredients:

- filtered water
- ginseng root
- lemon
- honey

Directions:

1. Measure 1–2 grams of ginseng root for each cup of tea you will prepare.
2. Boil 8 ounces of water per cup of tea.
3. Reduce the pot to a simmer and add the ginseng root.
4. Steep for 20–30 minutes.
5. Add honey and lemon to taste.
6. Strain the tea before drinking it (Teajoy Editorial Team, 2023).

California Poppy Tea

Teas made with the California poppy are particularly potent against insomnia fueled by anxiety. The best part about this plant is that all parts of it are medicinal.

Ingredients:

- small bundle of poppy parts
- 2 cups water

Directions:

1. Place the poppies in your cup.
2. Boil water and pour over the poppies.
3. Steep while covered for 20 minutes.
4. Strain and sweeten as desired before drinking (Rose, n.d.).

Passionflower Tea

Passionflower is a well-liked tea because of its slightly floral taste with a natural hint of sweetness.

Ingredients:

- dried passionflower

Directions:

1. Measure out 1 teaspoon of dried passionflower per cup of water.
2. Place the passionflower in a tea infuser or your teapot.
3. Pour boiling water over the passionflower.
4. Steep for 5–10 minutes.
5. Strain the tea before drinking (Akhtar, n.d.).

Magnolia Bark Tea

Magnolia bark has been used for centuries for its medicinal properties in Traditional Chinese medicine and Japanese traditional medicine. This recipe is a challenge to make due to the constraints of finding magnolia bark outside of Eastern cultures.

Ingredients:

- magnolia bark

Directions:

1. Measure your bark so that you have 2–4 twigs that measure 4 inches long or ¼ cup of loosely packed bark that you have peeled.
2. Rinse the bark with cold water.
3. Soak the bark in 8 cups of water for 30 minutes in the pot you will use to make the tea.
4. Bring the water to a boil and reduce to a simmer.
5. Cover and steep for 30 minutes to 2 hours.
6. Strain the tea, discarding the bark pieces (Superfoodly, 2020).

Sleepy Time Tea

From peppermint to lavender and passionflower, this tea gives you a taste of a ton of beneficial sleep-inducing herbs.

Ingredients:

- 1 part lavender and passionflower
- ¼ part valerian root
- 2 parts lemon balm
- 2 parts peppermint
- 3 parts chamomile
- 1 part catnip
- water

Directions:

1. Add all the herbs to a bowl and gently mix.
2. Place ½–1 tablespoon of the herbal blend into a tea infuser.
3. Boil the water.
4. Place the tea infuser in a mug and add the water.
5. Steep for 2–5 minutes.
6. Remove the infuser.
7. Enjoy warm (*How to Make Sleepy Time Tea*, n.d.).

Soothing Sleep Tea

This soothing tea recipe was created from ingredients that all have one important thing in common—they all support getting good sleep.

Ingredients:

- ½ cup dried lemon balm

- ¼ cup dried rose petals
- 1 cup dried chamomile
- 1 tbsp dried lavender

Directions:

1. Combine and blend all ingredients in a bowl. Between uses, keep it in a sealed container.
2. Steep 1 tablespoon of the herbal mixture in 8 ounces of boiling water for 5–15 minutes while covered.
3. Strain, sip, and relax (Szaro, 2022).

Sparkling Nightcap Tea

Catnip doesn't get the recognition it deserves among humans, as we most often recognize it as a feline stimulant. However, this tea capitalizes on its sedative qualities.

Ingredients:

- catnip tea
- boiling water
- sparkling water
- herbal iced tea
- organic honey
- valerian tincture

Directions:

1. Steep the catnip tea in boiling water for 30 seconds.

2. Move that teabag to sparkling water and steep for at least 10 minutes.
3. Add herbal iced tea, organic honey, and valerian tincture to the sparkling water.
4. Stir to blend before enjoying (Ali, 2021).

Sleepy Tea

This delicious herbal tea combines many excellent options for aiding in getting to sleep and having the perfect restful night.

Ingredients:

- 2 tbsp dried California poppy
- ¼ tbsp dried lemon balm
- 2 tbsp dried passionflower
- 2 tbsp dried rose petals
- 2 tbsp fennel seeds
- ¼ cup dried mint

Directions:

1. Combine poppy, lemon balm, passionflower, rose petals, fennel, and mint in a bowl. Stir to mix, then place in an airtight container.
2. Boil water.
3. Add 2 tablespoons of the herbal mixture into a heatproof container and pour 12 ounces of boiling water over it.

4. Steep for 5 minutes, strain, and serve (McGruther, 2021).

INTERACTIVE ELEMENT

When you're getting ready for bed and want to incorporate a sleep-inducing tea into your routine, there's nothing like a relaxing tea-drinking ritual to inspire you. While you can create a ritual that's designed specifically around you and your needs, here is a baseline idea you can use for your next cup of tea.

Start by selecting the ideal tea for relaxation and stress reduction to help you toward a peaceful night's sleep. With all the recipes we've just explored, you have many options. Ensure your selection speaks to you to get the most from the experience.

Consider where you will hold your ritual. It should be an environment that focuses on healing and relaxation. You'll need a space free of distractions and loud noises to focus on the mindfulness aspect of the ritual.

As you brew your tea, focus on the process. Breathe in the smells as your herbs steep in the boiling water. Listen to the sounds as you transfer them from their container to the cup. Be present in every action.

While your tea is steeping, consider a brief meditation to ensure your mind is in the right place. This will help further ease the day's tensions, allowing maximum relaxation. As you clear your thoughts, allow gratitude to enter your heart.

Roll the flavors around your mouth as you take each sip of your sleep-inducing tea. Take the time to recognize each herb and enjoy the experience as your body slowly decompresses and your mind slows down.

When you're finished drinking, pause for a moment to reflect on what you have to be grateful for. This practice can further remove the stressors from your mind, easing your tension and allowing for restful sleep.

One of the most common uses of medicinal herbs throughout history has been to aid in getting restful sleep. Modern science has frequently backed the efficacy of many of these popular herbal remedies. In the next chapter, we'll focus on another beneficial use of herbal teas: improving digestive health.

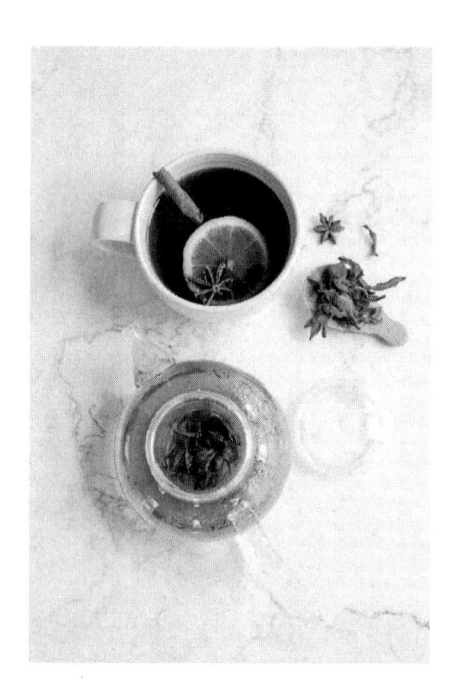

6

DISCOVER GINGER'S ZING WITH DIGESTIVE HEALTH-BOOSTING TEAS

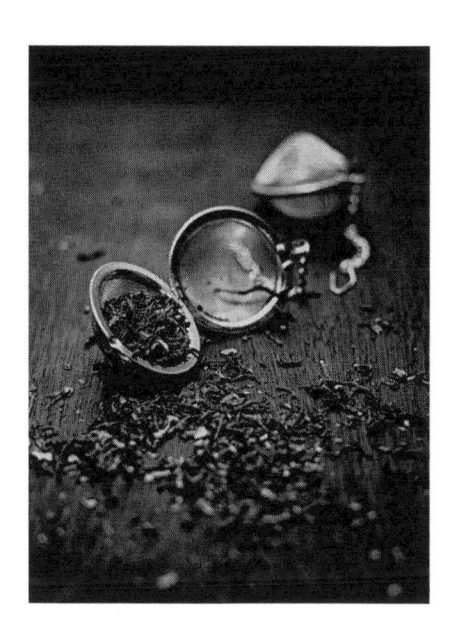

> *Tea is wealth itself, because there is nothing that cannot be lost, no problem that will not disappear, no burden that will not float away, between the first sip and the last.*
>
> — THE MINISTER OF LEAVES

Herbal tea can be a powerful tool for helping with digestive health concerns. Depending on your choice of herbs, you can target different symptoms to find the relief you need while supporting your overall gut health. While it may sound too good to be true, Martha found peppermint tea extremely helpful in her struggles with irritable bowel syndrome.

When she completed her research, she learned that peppermint offers the benefit of relaxing muscle tissues and can positively impact overall gut health. Because of this, she decided to brew her own peppermint herbal tea blend. Over time, she noticed a reduction in her symptoms, making it easier to cope with her condition naturally. As a bonus, the tea offered a wonderful flavor that she could enjoy day after day.

To understand how herbal teas can aid in digestive health and wellness, it's first important to establish a firm definition of what gut health is. We'll also consider the best herbs for gut health before exploring some fantastic digestive health-supporting tea recipes.

A GUIDE TO DIGESTIVE WELLNESS

When you set out to care for your digestive wellness, one of the most significant terms you will come across is "gut microbiome." While it sounds fancy, it simply refers to all the microorganisms within your gut or intestines. No matter who you are, you have around 200 different species living throughout your gastrointestinal tract, including viruses, bacteria, and fungi. Some microorganisms can be harmful; however, many are essential to proper gut health.

The more diversity in your gut microbiome, the more optimized your overall health will be. Research has demonstrated a strong link between your gut health and the following (Dix & Klein, 2018):

- gastrointestinal disorders
- cardiovascular disease
- autoimmune diseases
- endocrine disorders
- the immune system
- mental health
- cancer

Several different signs can identify an unhealthy digestive tract. One of the primary signs is an upset stomach. Symptoms of this issue can include bloating, gas, heartburn, constipation, and diarrhea. When your gut is balanced, you'll have less trouble digesting food and removing waste, dramatically reducing these symptoms.

If you generally consume a high-sugar diet, you likely have gut health problems. Excess sugar in your diet significantly decreases the number of good bacteria in your gut. In turn, this can produce inflammation throughout the body, which can cause certain conditions like cancer to develop.

When you gain or lose weight without having made significant changes to your diet or exercise habits, it's an indication that your gut health is no longer balanced. This imbalance can negatively impact your body's ability to properly perform several essential functions, including absorption of nutrients, fat storage, and blood sugar regulation. Weight loss can be due to bacterial overgrowth in the small intestine that causes malabsorption. In contrast, weight gain can directly result from insulin resistance or inflammation throughout the body.

Poor gut health is also related to chronic fatigue. When your gut bacteria are imbalanced, you may experience shortened sleep duration and fragmented sleep. This often results in chronic fatigue.

Your skin can also be affected by your gut health. Several skin conditions are related to the different types of bacteria naturally occurring in your gut. When they become imbalanced, it can lead to complications due to effects on the body's immune system.

Poor gut health can also lead to a poorly functioning immune system. When your gut isn't working correctly, you can experience increased systemic inflammation. As a result, you are at a greater risk of developing autoimmune diseases.

Finally, an imbalanced gut can lead to food intolerances, which are a direct result of having difficulties digesting specific types of foods. It's important to note that food allergies are not the same thing. When you have trouble digesting the foods that trigger these intolerances, you may experience abdominal pain, gas, bloating, diarrhea, and nausea.

If you're experiencing gut health problems, you can participate in a three-day gut reset. This special diet boosts your gut health by increasing the amount of beneficial bacteria in your large intestine. When you participate in a gut reset, you'll remove those foods that nurture the bad bacteria and promote inflammation, consume a range of prebiotic foods, and engage in several healthy practices that promote gut health.

On day one, your primary focus will be eliminating foods and drinks that cause inflammation. These include anything with added sugars, refined carbohydrates, and excessive saturated fats. You'll replace these foods with servings of your favorite fresh produce and healthy fats. You can also include complex carbohydrates to provide slow-burning energy for the day.

In addition to these healthy food choices, you'll need to drink enough water to ensure your body is fully hydrated. Observing your urine when you go to the bathroom is a quick check to see if you're on the right track. The ideal color is that of pale straw.

At the end of day one, ensure you have left yourself enough time to get a good night's sleep. As with many other things in your overall health, sleep or lack thereof can impact your gut health.

On day two, the focus will shift to adding foods rich in fiber. These food options will help feed the beneficial gut flora, helping boost your gut health. Note that this increase in fiber may cause some bloating or gas. If this becomes problematic, you can follow the day-one diet.

You'll also introduce regular exercise on this day. Not only does it promote healthy weight, but it can positively influence your microbiome, ensuring you have optimal gut health.

On day three, add some fermented foods to your diet. These foods are rich in probiotics. These foods are similar to high-fiber foods in that they may cause side effects. If you experience bloating and gas that does not go away, consider reducing your intake of fermented foods.

This is an opportune time to introduce mindfulness practices into your routine. By doing this, you can alleviate stress that can damage your gut microbiome. The more you relax, the better it is for your overall health and well-being.

Supporting your digestive health is essential to supporting your overall health. It provides three key benefits: immunity, sustenance, and emotional well-being. It might surprise you that your immunity begins deep within your gut. The immune system's inflammatory response is triggered here and is typically the result of the foods you eat. While your digestive system breaks down food into energy, if you have problems with nutrient breakdown or malabsorption, you may experience unpleasant symptoms. Your emotional health is also directly linked to your gut by the enteric nervous system (ENS). The ENS regulates digestion independently of the brain but constantly transmits information between the two areas of your body.

When you're ready to support your gut health, there are many steps you can take. One of the first things you should do is eat a healthy and balanced diet. Seek to eliminate as many processed, sugary, and fatty foods as possible from your diet. Consider increasing your fiber intake, which is linked to improved gut health. Additionally, be conscious about adding foods with the micronutrient polyphenols. When you eat like this, you will nourish your microbiome, which is an essential practice to support gut health.

Fermented foods are part of a three-day gut reset because of how beneficial they are to supporting the gut microbiome. They are all-natural probiotics that will help supplement the good bacteria already existing within your gut.

While it may seem unrelated, getting enough sleep is also essential to maintaining optimal gut health. You should strive to get seven to nine hours of uninterrupted sleep nightly. Anything less can result in gut health problems that contribute to even more complex sleeping issues.

When you exercise regularly, you can more easily maintain a healthy weight. This, in turn, helps with digestive problems. Daily physical activity keeps bowel activity regular, eliminating waste effectively from the body.

One of the most significant factors in developing poor gut health is experiencing a lot of stress. Chronic stress can take a severe toll on your entire body, but you can participate in activities that help reduce it. Consider any of the following:

- use an essential oil diffuser with calming essential oils
- practice a stress-relieving herbal tea ritual
- interact more with friends and family
- reduce alcohol consumption
- spend more time with a pet
- practice yoga
- meditate

Drinking water and staying hydrated are also key to maintaining gut health. Where you get the water from is just as important as how much you consume. You must ensure your water source is not tainted with infection-causing bacteria that can disrupt your gut health. Additionally, staying hydrated can help ease constipation issues and promote overall health.

As you identify food intolerances, eliminate those triggering foods from your diet. If you can avoid these foods, you'll be more likely to see an improvement in your gut health that improves your overall health.

You also need to take time to boost your immune system. You can do this by avoiding toxins whenever possible. This can include toxins in the water supply, common processed food items, and household and health and beauty products. Additionally, getting enough sun exposure on your skin will promote vitamin D production, boosting immune system health.

When you were growing up, your parents likely told you on more than one occasion to chew your food thoroughly and eat slowly. Turns out, this is more important than you could have imagined. By ensuring your food is broken down before it reaches your gut, you can facilitate the digestive process and prevent gut health problems.

You can also add prebiotics and probiotics to your daily routine for added gut health support. Prebiotics are food for good gut bacteria, while probiotics are live bacteria that benefit your microbiome. Choosing high-quality supplements is essential to getting the most out of them, so you may want to consult your physician for advice on which to purchase.

Eating garlic can improve the diversity of your microbiome. It will also boost your beneficial bacteria levels and improve your gut health. Collagen-rich foods, such as bone broth and salmon skin, are highly effective at boosting your gut health and should be added to your diet when possible.

NATURE'S HERBAL DIGESTIVE AIDS

Many herbs contain digestive-enhancing properties. These make excellent options for herbal remedies, including teas and tea blends.

Turmeric does a lot of wonderful things for your digestive health. Its primary benefit is its ability to reduce inflammation. It also increases the mucin content of the stomach and stops bleeding. With all three of these properties combined, turmeric is ideal for preventing ulcerations.

Consuming licorice root also increases mucin production. With this increased mucin, you'll enjoy better protection of the mucous membranes in your digestive tract.

Peppermint has a long history of effective use in individuals with IBS. It functions as a smooth muscle relaxant, which calms spasms and contractions in the gastrointestinal tract. It can also reduce gas, pain, and discomfort.

Ginger reduces muscle spasms and increases the production of digestive juices. The ingredients found in ginger help soothe the gut. They also promote increased peristalsis, which helps food move more efficiently through the intestines.

Cinnamon bark is a warming herb that can help stimulate a slow digestive system. Additionally, it can be used in cases of lost appetite, bloating, gas, and dyspepsia.

While chamomile has long been used for reducing stress and aiding sleep, it's also a great choice for the digestive system. It can help reduce the inflammation and cramps associated with chronic and acute gastric distress. Its antimicrobial and anti-inflammatory characteristics make it ideal for supporting the digestive system.

Lemon balm's traditional uses include aiding in reducing gas and bloating. Additionally, it may help reduce intestinal spasms and aid in regularity.

With its antioxidant properties, fennel helps heal damage from stomach ulcers while preventing more from developing. It also relieves constipation while promoting regularity and daily bowel movements

Gentian root contains bitter compounds, which increase the production of digestive acids and enzymes. Because of this, appetite is stimulated, and digestion is improved when gentian root is routinely consumed.

Angelica root contains a polysaccharide that increases healthy cells and blood vessels throughout the digestive tract. In turn, this helps prevent stomach damage. It can help fight the oxidative stress caused by ulcerative colitis and relieve constipation.

When you look at dandelions, you likely only see weeds. However, this herb can improve digestion by improving peristalsis. It can also help prevent ulcers by reducing inflammation and stomach acid production.

Senna is a digestive-supporting herb best used in moderation. It works on the smooth muscle of the intestine to promote bowel movements when you're experiencing constipation. However, it should not be consumed regularly, which can lead to diarrhea.

Marshmallow root contains antioxidant properties that aid in decreasing histamine, which is released during inflammation. It also helps promote mucus production to line the throat and stomach, protecting your digestive tract. It's an excellent choice for helping to prevent ulcers.

Black tea contains compounds that can aid in reducing indigestion by delaying gastric emptying. These compounds can help prevent stomach ulcers.

Wormwood promotes the production of digestive fluids, which causes a reduction in bloating and optimization of digestion.

Additionally, it may be able to kill certain parasites, further promoting a healthy digestive tract.

DIGESTIVE HEALTH-SUPPORTING TEA RECIPES

If you want to boost your digestive health, teas are a great option. Let's explore some excellent digestive health-supporting tea recipes you can easily make in your kitchen.

Gentian Root Tea

While the Gentiana family of plants can be found in many locations worldwide and has many medicinal properties, the roots of the plants are the focus of herbal tea recipes like this one.

Ingredients:

- 2 g dried gentian root
- 8 oz water

Directions:

1. Boil the water.
2. Place the gentian root in a teapot.
3. Pour the water over the root.
4. Place the lid on the teapot and steep for 10–15 minutes.
5. Strain and drink before eating (Bibe, 2020).

Senna Tea

This senna tea recipe is ideal for soothing constipation issues. Be careful not to consume it too often, or you may experience diarrhea.

Ingredients:

- 1 tsp dried senna leaves
- 8 oz water

Directions:

1. Boil the water and pour over the senna leaves.
2. Cover and steep for 10–15 minutes.
3. Strain before drinking (Bibe, 2020).

Angelica Root Tea

You can drink this tea when you're experiencing inflammatory side effects from ulcerative colitis or have a case of constipation.

Ingredients:

- 1 tbsp dried angelica root
- 8 oz water

Directions:

1. Boil the water and pour over the angelica root.

2. Cover and steep the tea for 10–15 minutes.
3. Strain before drinking (Bibe, 2020).

Marshmallow Root Tea

Marshmallow root tea is excellent for reducing the development of ulcers that nonsteroidal anti-inflammatory drugs (NSAIDs) can cause.

Ingredients:

- 1 tbsp dried marshmallow root
- 8 oz water

Directions:

1. Boil the water and pour over the marshmallow root.
2. Cover and steep for 10–15 minutes.
3. Strain the marshmallow root from the tea before drinking (Bibe, 2020).

Dandelion Tea

Dandelion is an easy-to-use herb; you can use any part of the plant to make this tea.

Ingredients:

- 1 tsp dandelion (can use flowers, stems, or roots)
- 8 oz water

Directions:

1. Place the dandelion in a cup and pour boiling water over it.
2. Steep while covered for 10–15 minutes.
3. Strain the tea and enjoy it (Bibe, 2020).

Cinnamon Apple Tea

To get the most out of this tea blend, it's best to use organic apples. You can buy them dried or dry them yourself.

Ingredients:

- ½ tbsp crushed cinnamon bark
- 1 tbsp dried apple pieces

Instructions:

1. Combine the cinnamon bark and apple pieces in a container and mix well.
2. Place 1 teaspoon of the herbal mixture in a cup.
3. Pour one cup of boiling water over the mixture.
4. Steep for 5–10 minutes.
5. Strain and enjoy (*8 Simple*, 2020).

Herbal Chai Tea

Unlike regular chai, this herbal tea has no caffeine, ensuring your digestive tract doesn't get any unwanted stimulation. This recipe makes 4–5 servings.

Ingredients:

- 2 in. crushed cinnamon bark
- ½–1 tsp crushed cardamom
- 4 spoons rooibos tea
- 1 tsp ginger powder
- ½–1 tsp cloves

Directions:

1. Combine all ingredients, mixing well, and store in an airtight container.
2. Add 1 teaspoon of the herbal mixture to a cup.
3. Boil 1 cup of water and pour over the herbs.
4. Steep for 5–10 minutes.
5. Strain before serving (*8 Simple*, 2020).

Fennel Tea

You can drink this tea daily to help you remain regular. It's also great for healing ulcers.

Ingredients:

- 1 tsp dried fennel root or fennel seeds

- 8 oz water

Directions:

1. Place the fennel in a cup.
2. Pour boiling water over it.
3. Steep for 10–15 minutes.
4. Strain the tea before drinking (Bibe, 2020).

Cardamom Ginger Chai Tea

While this tea is a bit spicy, it packs a powerful medicinal punch. You can adjust the cardamom and ginger to your liking.

Ingredients:

- 1 cup water
- small piece of ginger, grated
- several cardamom pods
- 1–2 tbsp unflavored black tea leaves
- 1 cup milk
- sweetener of choice

Directions:

1. Bring water, ginger, and cardamom to a boil.
2. Add the tea leaves.
3. Remove the tea leaves promptly after 30 seconds.
4. Add the milk and allow it to come to a gentle boil.

5. Remove the chai from the heat when the milk starts to bubble over.
6. Strain the chai into a cup.
7. Add a neutral sweetener (Modern African Table, n.d.)

Clove and Cinnamon Tea

Combining cloves and cinnamon offers an incredible boost to your digestive health.

Ingredients:

- 1 tsp cinnamon
- 1 cup water
- 4–5 cloves

Directions:

1. Combine all ingredients in a saucepan and bring to a boil.
2. Continue boiling for 3–5 minutes.
3. Reduce hit to simmer for 10 minutes.
4. Cool to your desired temperature, strain, and enjoy (Foods4Health, n.d.).

Easy Homemade Tea for Digestion

This recipe is a great option for preparing in bulk, as it can be stored on the pantry shelf for up to six months.

Ingredients:

- 1 tbsp dried ginger pieces
- 2 tbsp fenugreek seeds
- 2 tbsp coriander seeds
- 2 tbsp fennel seeds
- 1 tbsp cumin seeds

Directions:

1. Combine all ingredients, mixing well, and store in a tightly sealed container in your pantry.
2. For each cup brewed, use 1 teaspoon of the herbal blend.
3. Combine herbal blend and water in a saucepan and bring to a boil.
4. Reduce to a simmer and cover.
5. Simmer for 20 minutes.
6. Strain the tea before serving.
7. Add sweetener if desired (Perry, 2021).

After-Dinner Belly-Soothing Tea

If you've ever experienced that feeling after dinner where you've overeaten and your belly is bloated and uncomfortable, this recipe has the soothing solution you need.

Ingredients:

- 1 tsp fennel seeds, lightly crushed

- ½ tsp dried cut ginger pieces
- 1 tsp dried chamomile flowers
- 1 tsp dried peppermint leaves
- 8 oz boiling water
- honey to taste

Directions:

1. Combine fennel, ginger, chamomile, and peppermint in a teapot.
2. Pour boiling water over the herbs.
3. Cover and steep for 10 minutes.
4. Strain and sweeten as desired (Han, 2020).

The Ultimate Stomach-Soothing Tea

Nourishing the gut is key to maintaining balance in your overall health and wellness. This recipe can help you do that.

Ingredients:

- 1 part marshmallow root
- ¼ part peppermint
- ½ part calendula
- 1 part chamomile
- 1 part fennel

Directions:

1. Combine all ingredients, mix well, and store in a tightly sealed container.
2. To brew, combine 1 cup of boiling water with 1 teaspoon of herbal tea.
3. Steep for 10 minutes while covered.
4. Strain the herbs from the tea before enjoying it (Saba, 2019).

Gut-Healing Tea

This tea offers a variety of benefits, including relieving ulcers, acid reflux, and leaky gut.

Ingredients:

- 1 part dried marshmallow leaf or flower
- 2 parts dried marshmallow root
- sprinkle of dried rose petals
- 1 part dried plantain leaf
- 1 part dried fennel seed

Optional ingredients per cup:

- 1–2 cardamom pods
- pinch of licorice root
- 1–2 cinnamon sticks
- 3–5 whole cloves
- 1 star anise pod

Directions:

1. Add all herbs to an airtight container, mix well, and store in a cool, dark location.
2. Place 2 or more heaping teaspoonfuls of herbal mixture in a 32-ounce container.
3. Cover the herbal mixture with hot water.
4. Cover the container and steep for several hours. You can also let it sit overnight.
5. Strain the tea.
6. Drink over 1–2 days (Groves, 2019).

Good Digestion Tea

You'll immediately love the decadent flavor combination when you prepare this tea recipe.

Ingredients:

- 3½ oz dried peppermint
- 3½ oz dried chamomile
- 1 oz orange peel
- ½ oz cinnamon
- ½ oz ginger
- 1 oz licorice

Directions:

1. Combine all ingredients, mix well, and store in an airtight container.

2. Place 8 tablespoons of the herbal blend in a teapot and add 1 quart of boiling water.
3. Cover and steep for 15–20 minutes.
4. Strain the herbs before drinking.
5. Sweeten as desired and drink 1 cup as needed (Martha Stewart Test Kitchen, 2019).

Stomach-Soother Tea

This easy-to-make calming tea is perfect for those with digestive troubles.

Ingredients:

- pinch of dried ginger
- ½ tsp fennel seeds
- 2 tsp mint leaf

Directions:

1. Combine and mix ingredients in a cup.
2. Pour boiling water over the herbs.
3. Steep while covered for 5 minutes.
4. Strain and enjoy (Wells, 2012).

Best Digestive Tea Recipe

For a beneficial boost to your gut health, drink this tea right after eating.

Ingredients:

- 3 cups water
- 1 tsp dried lemon balm leaves
- 1 tsp dried peppermint leaves
- 1 tsp fenugreek
- 1 cinnamon stick
- ½ lemon slice
- 2 tsp honey

Optional ingredients:

- 1 in. fresh turmeric, sliced
- 1 in. fresh ginger, sliced

Directions:

1. Combine water, lemon balm, peppermint, and fenugreek in a saucepan, cover, boil, and remove from the heat.
2. Add the rest of the ingredients except for the honey. Steep for 5–10 minutes while covered.
3. Strain the herbs from the tea and add the sweetener before serving (Lilly, 2023).

Soothing Marshmallow Rose Tea

If you need a soothing solution for your digestive tract, consider trying this herbal tea.

Ingredients:

- 1 tsp fenugreek part organic sweet cinnamon powder
- 1 part organic sweet cinnamon chips
- 3 parts organic marshmallow root
- filtered, distilled, or spring water
- 2 parts organic rose buds
- raw, local honey

Directions:

1. Using a pint-sized jar, measure the herbs to fill the jar one-third full.
2. Fill the remainder of the jar with cool water.
3. Refrigerate the jar overnight.
4. The following morning, strain the tea.
5. Add honey to taste and enjoy (Heidi, 2022).

Herbal Digestive Tea Blend

While this tea is great for digestion, you may drink it for the flavor alone. If you have concerns about high blood pressure, you can substitute stevia leaf for the licorice root.

Ingredients:

- 1 part dried goldenrod leaves and flowers
- 1 part hawthorn berries, whole
- ½ part dried licorice root
- ½ part dried ginger root

- 1 part dried lemongrass

Directions:

1. Combine all ingredients and store them in an airtight container.
2. Combine 1 tablespoon with 8 ounces of hot water when brewing your tea.
3. Steep for 5–15 minutes while covered.
4. Strain before sipping (de la Forêt, 2016).

Orange-Spiced Black Tea

This tea blend is all about the flavors and the beautiful presentation. You get the luxury of a fine-tasting tea while reaping digestive health benefits.

Ingredients:

- 1 tsp orange extract
- 1 cup Assam tea
- a few dried orange slices
- 1 tbsp cardamom pods, lightly crushed
- 1 tbsp rainbow peppercorns
- 1 tbsp cinnamon chips

Directions:

1. Place the orange extract in a quart-sized glass jar. Shake until the extract thoroughly covers the inside of the jar.

2. Add the tea, orange slices, cardamom, peppercorns, and cinnamon chips. Shake well.
3. Allow this mixture to sit for a day to soak up the orange extract.
4. When brewing, use 1 teaspoon of the herbal blend for 8 ounces of hot water.
5. Steep for 3–5 minutes.
6. Strain before adding your choice of milk or cream and honey or sugar. You can also drink it plain (de la Forêt, 2016).

INTERACTIVE ELEMENT

Stress and anxiety are leading contributors to poor gut health. Minimizing their influence is essential to boosting your good bacteria, managing the bad bacteria, and enjoying a smoothly operating digestive system. Incorporating a tea ritual into your daily activities can help soothe stress and anxiety and help accomplish this goal.

While you'll be focusing on the act of the ritual as a method of destressing, you'll want to select a tea that optimizes digestive health. Consider your current symptoms and which herbs can benefit you the most.

Once you have your tea selected, it's time to choose the time and location of your ceremony. It's best to establish at least 30 minutes to give yourself. Self-care is essential to your health and well-being, and cutting it short benefits no one.

Place your tea into your special ritual cup and brew your chosen tea. After it has steeped, head to your ritual location. Sit comfortably and slowly sip and savor your tea. As the flavors roll across your tongue, imagine how the herbs will journey through your body, healing you.

Ensure that every action you take is done with deliberation. Calm your breathing and clear your mind, focusing on nothing but the act of drinking the tea until it's gone. Repeat the ritual at the same time daily for the best results.

Many different herbs can positively impact your digestive health. Moreover, most of them taste fantastic when brewed in an herbal tea blend, making them more palatable than other options. In the next chapter, we'll focus on how to use herbs to boost immunity.

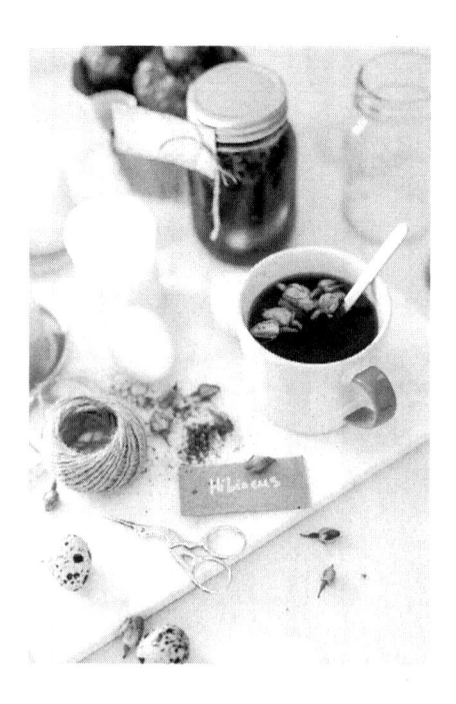

7

BOOST YOUR IMMUNITY WITH ECHINACEA ELIXIRS AND OTHER TEAS

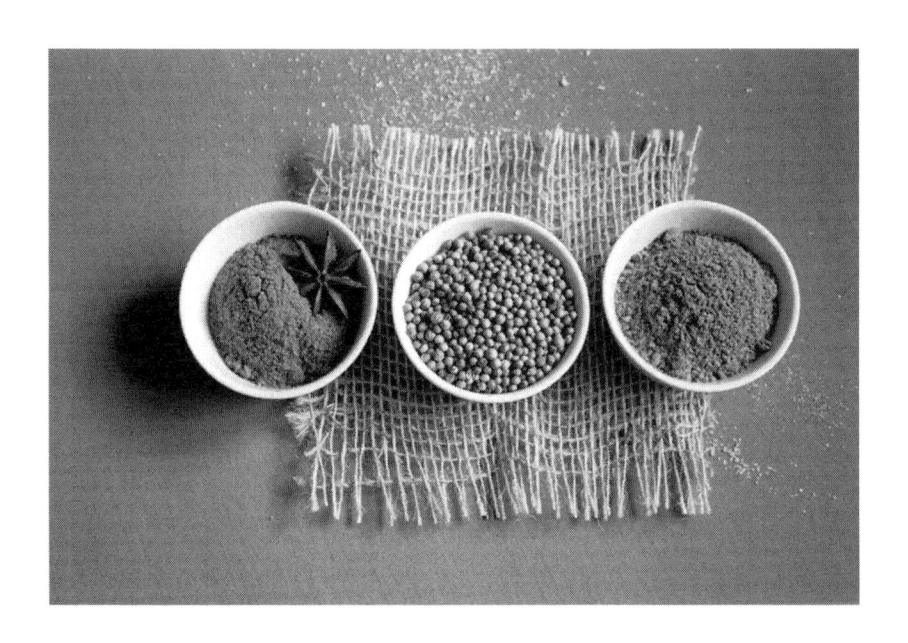

> *There are those who love to get dirty and fix things. They drink coffee at dawn, beer after work. And those who stay clean, just appreciate things. At breakfast, they have milk and juice at night. There are those who do both, they drink tea.*
>
> — GARY SNYDER

Drinking herbal teas focusing on immunity is a great way to boost your overall health and wellness. Herbs contain various components linked to better health, which makes these tea blends so potent. Consider an immune-boosting herbal tea if you experience seasonal illnesses or other conditions.

Carl often suffered from seasonal colds and sought a way to help boost his immune system to ward off the impending sickness in the fall and winter. After finding several recipes that offered the benefits he needed, he incorporated drinking them into his daily routine. Over time, he noticed an improvement in his general well-being and a reduction in the number of times he experienced sickness.

To understand how herbal teas can benefit your immune system, it's important to first understand how to build stronger immunity. We'll start this chapter with a look at the science behind this.

THE SCIENCE BEHIND BUILDING A STRONG IMMUNE SYSTEM

Your immune system is a crucial piece of your health and well-being. It is your body's source of protection from disease-causing microorganisms. A healthy immune system protects you from many threats, ranging from the common cold to more severe conditions like cancer. It is an elaborate system impacted by many factors. You can help support your immune system by taking several different actions, including getting regular vaccinations, eating a healthy diet, and avoiding certain bad habits.

Smoking is one of those bad habits you should avoid or stop if you've already started. It can compromise your immune system, making you more susceptible to immune system problems, including rheumatoid arthritis. Additionally, your body will have a harder time fighting off diseases as it works to protect you from the toxins generated by smoking.

Because most of your immune system can be found in your gut, keeping your gut health optimal is essential. You need to fuel your body with a healthy diet rich in fruits and vegetables to do this. These foods will provide the necessary vitamin C and antioxidants to help your immune system do its job.

Getting regular exercise will also increase the activity of your immune system. Staying active increases the circulation of the key players in your immune system—white blood cells and antibodies. Because their movement will increase, they'll be better able to identify and hone in on those threats to your health. Additionally, staying active reduces the production of your stress hormone, which can also aid in preventing sickness.

Maintaining a healthy weight is another key way to support your immune system. Obesity and impaired immunity are closely linked. Additionally, being obese can result in decreased effectiveness of some vaccines, including the influenza vaccine.

Alcohol should be consumed in moderation. Excessive alcohol consumption is linked to weakened immune systems. If you drink alcohol, you don't necessarily have to stop. However, you do need to monitor how much and how often you drink.

We've come to another important health and wellness aspect that relies on adequate sleep. The immune system cannot function optimally if your body is overtired. You must regularly get seven to nine hours of uninterrupted sleep nightly to ensure your body has the energy to fight off illness.

During the peak of the COVID-19 pandemic, we were frequently reminded of the need to wash our hands regularly and thoroughly. This is a practice to be incorporated into your daily activities, no matter the social circumstances. If you go to the store, there are millions of germs you will come into contact with, especially on your shopping cart. At work, you may share a pen with someone and pass germs. An innocent handshake could spread illness. All these are excellent reasons to wash your hands for a solid 20 seconds with warm water and soap frequently throughout your day.

Meat can contain bacteria and other pathogens that must be cooked off. The only way to do this is to thoroughly cook it all the way through. While many enjoy their meats on the lighter side of done, it can be risky to consume it this way. To ensure your immune system stays healthy, you need to ensure your meat is well done.

Reducing stress is crucial to protecting your immune system. The more stress you experience, the more cortisol is produced. Cortisol suppresses the immune system's function, making it easier for you to get sick. On top of that, stress makes you less likely to focus on other healthy habits.

Vaccinations help boost your immune system by teaching it about the illnesses they are made for. Staying on top of your vaccination schedule can ensure your immune system will be prepared for whatever comes your way.

When you choose the foods you eat, consider those rich in antioxidants and vitamin C. Antioxidants protect the body from oxidative stress, boosting the immune system. Vitamin C supports the immune system so that it can ward off illness.

Keeping your good bacteria healthy and happy is essential to promoting your immune system. Supporting those bacteria with prebiotics is a great way to do this. You can take a supplement or include asparagus, green bananas, or fermented foods in your diet.

Garlic is another natural choice for boosting the immune system. If you can, the best way to consume garlic is by eating half of a raw clove daily. If you can't stomach that, try roasting it.

A GUIDE TO IMMUNE-BOOSTING HERBS

Another great way to boost your immune system is using herbs with immune-boosting properties. Luckily, there are a ton of different options to choose from.

Astragalus is a commonly used herb in Traditional Chinese medicine (TCM). It's primarily used as an adaptogen, which helps protect your body from disease and stress. Additionally, it can be used in herbal blends to help treat the common cold and boost the immune system.

Black elderberry is an excellent source of antioxidants. Because of this, it provides excellent immune system support. It gets its rich, deep purple coloring from its high concentration of anthocyanins, which are also responsible for the herb's immune-boosting properties.

Someone has likely recommended or mentioned echinacea to you at one time or another. It is widely used during cold and flu season. It contains compounds that help shorten the duration of a cold and flu, helping to ease associated symptoms, such as sore throat and fever.

Ginger is another traditionally used herb that has immune-boosting benefits. It offers antioxidant, analgesic, and anti-inflammatory benefits that improve immune system function. In turn, this can lead to better protection against chronic conditions.

While goldenseal offers beneficial support for mucus tissues throughout your respiratory and digestive systems, it is an endangered plant due to overharvesting. It should only be used ethically and sustainably when you need to boost mucus membrane function to support your immune system.

Native Americans traditionally used grindelia for respiratory health. If your respiratory tract is irritated, grindelia can provide support and relief. Its flowers secrete a sticky sap that benefits the tissues within the respiratory system.

Maitake is a mushroom commonly used in TCM and Japanese traditional medicine. It contains beta-glucans, which are relied on to support overall health and wellness.

Olive leaf is a great source of antioxidants to protect your body from exposure to free radicals. In addition, it also supports a healthy body temperature and beneficial levels of immune cells. This helps promote good immune, cardiovascular, and glycemic health.

You probably use oregano a lot in the kitchen, but you may not know that this herb is highly beneficial to your immune system. It offers antiviral, antifungal, and antibacterial properties that help support an overall healthy immune response. In addition, it contains volatile oils that promote healthy respiratory function.

Reishi is another type of mushroom used in TCM and is considered an adaptogen. Like maitake, it contains beta-glucans, which are responsible for supporting a strong immune response.

Turmeric has long been used in the Ayurvedic tradition of medicine. Its primary active component is curcumin, which has antioxidant and anti-inflammatory properties. Curcumin is highly beneficial for improving oxidative stress markers.

Cinnamon is a well-rounded herb with many excellent properties, including antioxidant, anti-inflammatory, antifungal, and antibacterial benefits. Adding this herb to your diet can give your immune system that much-needed boost.

Peppermint is an herb containing various flavonoids, promoting immune health. Additionally, it is a menthol source, offering analgesic and anesthetic benefits.

Paprika supports the immune system with its powerful combination of vitamins A and C. Vitamin C protects your body from free radicals and promotes the health of immune cells, while vitamin A aids in immune system development and the regulation of immune responses.

While green tea is not an herbal option, it can benefit the immune system. It contains catechin and quercetin, which are both antioxidants. Catechin helps protect your body from oxidative stress, reducing the risk of getting an infection or disease. Additionally, it can protect you from contracting the flu. Quercetin is beneficial at fighting off viruses responsible for the common cold.

Black tea, one of the most commonly drank teas worldwide, has immune-boosting properties. It encourages the release of T cells responsible for fighting off various types of infections. Additionally, it contains the immune-boosting minerals potassium and manganese.

White tea is the least popular choice when green and black teas are also on the menu. However, it is a better source of antioxidants. It also offers antibacterial properties. This combination of benefits helps your body fight off infections while boosting your immune system.

Licorice root is great as a tea when you're sick. It helps to soothe a sore throat and offers a refreshingly sweet taste. It has antiviral and antibacterial properties that support a healthy immune system and ward off colds and the flu.

Hibiscus is an excellent source of vitamin C. You can even meet your daily requirement of this essential vitamin with three cups of hibiscus tea. You can effectively boost your immune system health with this herb.

IMMUNE-BOOSTING TEA RECIPES

With so many immune-boosting herbs to choose from, you can positively impact your overall health by creating some delicious tea recipes. I have several great options to share with you.

Cumin Coriander Fennel Tea

This tea recipe comes from the Ayurvedic tradition and provides a broad-spectrum focus on health and well-being.

Ingredients:

- 1 tsp cumin seeds
- 1 tsp coriander

- 1 tsp fennel

Optional ingredients:

- ½ tsp fresh ginger, grated
- pinch of black pepper
- pinch of cardamom
- holy basil leaves

Directions:

1. Combine ingredients in 6 cups of water.
2. Boil, strain, and serve.

This tea can be sipped throughout the day. If you'd like, add honey and a pinch of lemon once it reaches a lukewarm temperature. Do not add these two ingredients when hot (Herman, 2020).

Echinacea, Chamomile, and Raspberry Tea

All three of these ingredients are well-known for their immunity-boosting properties, giving you a powerful punch in every cup.

Ingredients:

- raspberry leaf
- chamomile
- echinacea

Directions:

1. Combine the desired amount of each ingredient in a tea infuser in your favorite teacup.
2. Pour hot water over the infuser.
3. Steep to your desired strength.
4. Remove the infuser and enjoy your tea (Herman, 2020).

Ginger, Turmeric, and Black Pepper Tea

This tea is the perfect combination to reduce inflammation and boost the immune system.

Ingredients:

- 1 pinch black pepper
- 1 pinch turmeric
- 1 pinch ginger

Directions:

1. Combine the three ingredients with 1 cup of water in a small saucepan and boil.
2. Pour into a cup and drink (Herman, 2020).

Lemon Cinnamon Tea

It's important to note that you should not add milk to this tea, as it will reduce its immune-boosting effects.

Ingredients:

- 1 cup green tea
- ½ tsp lemon juice
- 1 cinnamon stick
- 1 tsp honey

Directions:

1. Prepare your green tea.
2. Add the remaining ingredients and enjoy (Herman, 2020).

Lemon Pepper Tea

If you're looking for a way to boost your natural resistance and fight fatigue, this tea has what you need.

Ingredients:

- black pepper
- turmeric
- lemon
- honey

Directions:

1. Combine pepper and turmeric in a cup.
2. Add boiling water.
3. Squeeze in lemon.

4. Add honey to taste and enjoy (Jaswal, 2021).

Turmeric Tea

Turmeric tea is the perfect source of antioxidants to give your immune system a much-needed boost.

Ingredients:

- ½ tsp ginger, peeled and chopped
- ½ tsp turmeric tea, squashed
- natural sweetener
- lemon juice

Directions:

1. Boil 2 full glasses of water.
2. Reduce the heat and add the turmeric and ginger.
3. Steep for 5–7 minutes.
4. Strain into your serving cups.
5. Add sweetener and lemon juice to taste (Jaswal, 2021).

Immunity-Boosting Spiced Tea

This tea will help your immune system ward off infections, as it contains a generous helping of anti-inflammatory and antimicrobial benefits.

Ingredients:

- 1 cardamom pod, crushed

- 1 in. cinnamon stick
- handful of tulsi leaves
- 1 tbsp ginger, grated
- 2 peppercorns
- 1 star anise
- 2 cloves
- 1 tbsp unpasteurized honey

Directions:

1. Combine all ingredients except the honey in a pan.
2. Add 1 quart of water and boil for 30 minutes.
3. Drink ¼ cup with a dash of honey (Momaya, 2020).

Hot Lemonade

The combination of ginger, garlic, and cinnamon in this drink lends a powerful boost to the immune system and helps fight disease.

Ingredients:

- 4 cups water
- 4 fresh garlic cloves, chopped
- 1 tsp fresh ginger, grated
- 1 in. cinnamon stick
- 1 tbsp mint leaves
- juice of 1 lemon
- 2 tbsp raw honey

Directions:

1. Boil the water and add all other ingredients except the honey.
2. Steep for 30 minutes.
3. Strain into a glass.
4. Add honey to taste and enjoy (Momaya, 2020).

Spice Ginger Tea

When the winter blues have you down and you need to ward off the cold season, this tea is perfect.

Ingredients:

- cardamom
- cinnamon
- pepper
- ginger
- honey
- clove

Directions:

1. Combine the spices and ginger slices in the sieve of a kettle.
2. Fill the kettle with water.
3. Bring the kettle to a boil, then reduce to a simmer.
4. Simmer for 7–10 minutes.
5. Serve in individual cups with honey (Azmanov, 2017).

Cinnamon Ginger Turmeric Tea

Not only does this tea offer excellent immune-boosting assistance, but it also tastes great.

Ingredients:

- ginger
- black pepper
- agave syrup
- cinnamon
- turmeric
- lemon
- 17 oz water

Directions:

1. Peel and grate the ginger into a medium-sized pan.
2. Add remaining ingredients.
3. Pour in water.
4. Heat for approximately 4 minutes until steam rises from the pan. Whisk continuously to help the turmeric and cinnamon dissolve.
5. Strain and serve with fresh lemon and ginger (Ferko, 2020).

Cinnamon Sore Throat Tea

This tea is perfect for providing the comfort you need when you have an aching sore throat.

Ingredients:

- 1 cup milk
- ½ tsp ginger, powdered and ground
- ½ tsp cinnamon, ground
- 1 tbsp mild-tasting honey

Directions:

1. Scald milk in a saucepan until hot but not boiling.
2. Stir in the remaining ingredients, blending completely.
3. Sip slowly to soothe your throat (Debi, 2015).

Medicine Ball Copycat Tea

This recipe takes the best flavors of a popular chain's cold-busting tea, allowing you to make it at home. This is the perfect solution when you feel that cold weather is coming on.

Ingredients:

- 1 bag Teavana Peach Tranquility Tea
- 1 bag Teavana Jade Citrus Mint Tea
- 1 cup lemonade
- 1 cup hot water
- honey to taste

Directions:

1. Heat lemonade and add to a 16-ounce mug.

2. Add hot water and stir.
3. Add both tea bags and steep for 3–5 minutes.
4. Add honey as desired (Carrie, 2022).

Goji Berry Tea

Goji berries are another great resource for boosting your immune system. They offer a great taste and can be used in many ways, including this tea recipe.

Ingredients:

- 4 cups hot water
- 6–8 tbsp dried goji berries

Directions:

1. Pour hot water over the berries.
2. Steep 20 minutes.
3. Scoop into cups, splitting the berries between each serving (Zen, 2022).

Warm Honey Green Tea

You can enjoy the warming benefits of this immune-boosting tea on a cold night, although you'll find it delicious and supportive any time of year.

Ingredients:

- 4 cups water

- 4 lemon peel strips
- 4 orange peel strips
- 4 green tea bags
- 2 tsp honey
- 4 lemon slices

Directions:

1. Combine water and lemon and orange peels in a medium saucepan.
2. Bring to a boil and reduce heat.
3. Simmer for 10 minutes, keeping uncovered.
4. Remove the peels with a slotted spoon and discard.
5. Place green tea bags in a teapot and add the simmering water.
6. Cover and steep according to the directions on the packaging.
7. Remove the tea bags, squeeze gently, and discard.
8. Add honey and stir.
9. Pour the tea into four cups and garnish with lemon slices (EatingWell Test Kitchen, n.d.).

Immune-Boosting Ginger and Turmeric Tea

No matter the season, this tea is perfect for helping build up your immune system.

Ingredients:

- ½ tsp fresh turmeric, grated

- ½ tsp fresh ginger, grated
- pinch black pepper
- 2 cups water

Directions:

1. Combine all ingredients in a small saucepan and bring to a boil.
2. Turn off the heat and steep for 5 minutes.
3. Strain into a mug and enjoy immediately (Hu, 2020).

Ginger Lemon Tea

Enjoy the soothing benefits of this tea blend while you boost your immunity. The combination of lemon, ginger, and green tea offers excellent benefits to help keep sickness at bay.

Ingredients:

- 6 cups water
- 2 in. fresh ginger, peeled and thinly sliced
- 8 strips lemon peel
- 3 green tea bags
- 5 lemon slices
- 1 tbsp sugar substitute

Directions:

1. Combine water, ginger, and lemon peels. Bring to a boil.

2. Reduce heat and simmer for 10 minutes.
3. Remove the ginger and lemon peels with a slotted spoon and discard.
4. Place the green tea bags in a teapot and add the simmering water.
5. Cover and steep for 1–3 minutes.
6. Remove the tea bags, squeeze gently, and discard.
7. Serve immediately with lemon slices and sugar substitute (EatingWell Test Kitchen, 2023).

Immune Booster Tea

This tea is great for supporting your immune system but can also be used as an anti-inflammatory support before working out.

Ingredients:

- 3 cups water
- 1 in. fresh turmeric root
- 2 cloves garlic, chopped
- 1 in. fresh ginger
- handful moringa leaves
- handful cerasee leaves
- sweetener to taste

Directions:

1. Boil water in a large pot.
2. Add turmeric, garlic, and ginger.

3. Reduce heat and simmer for 10–15 minutes.
4. Remove from heat.
5. Add moringa and cerasee leaves.
6. Cover and steep for 10 minutes.
7. Strain before serving (Blackwood, 2021).

Herbal Immune Tea

No one wants to suffer through a cold or flu. This herbal tea can help boost your immune system to shorten the duration of symptoms and protect you from the viruses that cause these illnesses.

Ingredients:

- 4–5 cups water
- 1 tbsp orange peel
- 1 tbsp elderberries
- 2 tsp licorice root
- 1 tbsp echinacea
- honey to taste

Directions:

1. Combine water and herbs in a pot.
2. Bring to a boil and reduce to a simmer
3. Continue simmering for 30 minutes.
4. Strain and sweeten as desired.
5. Drink 1 cup daily (Cohen, 2020).

Herbal Cold-Remedy Tea

If you're on the hunt for a home remedy that takes a shot at cold and flu symptoms, try this tea recipe on for size.

Ingredients:

- 2 in. fresh ginger, peeled
- 1 tbsp ground turmeric
- 1 cup raw honey
- 2 halved lemons, sliced thinly and seeded
- 1 halved orange, sliced thinly and seeded
- 2 halved limes, sliced thinly and seeded
- hot water

Directions:

1. Use a mortar and pestle to grind the ginger into a paste.
2. Mix ginger, turmeric, and honey in a large bowl.
3. Stir in fruit slices and mix well.
4. For one serving, combine 2 tablespoons of the tea blend with hot water in a mug and stir to blend.
5. Store the remaining tea blend in an airtight container (Kelly, 2020).

Hippy Cold-Care Tea

This tea blend is derived from folk medicine, used initially to reduce fevers.

Ingredients:

- 1 part yarrow flowers and leaves
- 1 part peppermint leaves
- 1 part elderflower

Directions:

1. Measure your herbs for the desired total product.
2. Place 4–6 tablespoons of the herbal mixture in a heatproof quart-sized container.
3. Fill the container to the top with boiling water.
4. Steep uncovered for 30–45 minutes.
5. Strain the herbs before drinking.
6. Refrigerate any remaining tea and reheat as you want more (Anthis, 2014).

Headache-Relief Tea

Headaches are a common problem when sickness rolls around. This tea is perfect for relieving that tension.

Ingredients:

- ¼ part lemon balm
- 1 part chamomile
- ¼ part lavender
- 1 part basil leaf

Directions:

1. Measure the herbs to produce the total desired tea.
2. Place 4–6 tablespoons of the herbal mixture in a heatproof quart-sized container.
3. Fill the container to the top with boiling water.
4. Steep uncovered for 30–45 minutes.
5. Strain the tea before drinking.
6. Refrigerate any remaining tea. Reheat servings as you want more (Anthis, 2014).

INTERACTIVE ELEMENT

Stress and anxiety are often overwhelming aspects of our lives. Practicing mindfulness can be challenging because we frequently feel we lack the time to do it. However, suppose you enjoy drinking tea and do it routinely. In that case, it's easy to incorporate a few minutes of mindful activity into your daily routine to help ease the onset of stress and anxiety. Additionally, you can take the opportunity to add immune-boosting herbs to get both benefits at once.

No matter which calming, soothing, and healing tea you select, the purpose of your tea-drinking activity is to encourage a reduction in stress and anxiety. To do this, you will need a quiet place. You can be alone or with like-minded individuals who want to share in the moment.

Start by consciously boiling your water and steeping your tea. While you wait, reflect on something positive in your life. This will help ease some of the worry that is weighing you down. As you reflect, embrace your gratefulness and let it fill you.

When your tea is ready, move to your quiet place and take the first soothing sip. As it fills your mouth, relish the flavors as they swirl around your tongue. Feel the healing powers as the tea moves from your mouth toward your stomach. Enjoy how it warms you. Be present in every moment.

While you continue drinking your tea, reflect on the positives in your life, as this will give you meaning and purpose for your day. Whenever something negative tries to force its way into your mind, redirect your thoughts toward what you are grateful for. Continue this until your tea is gone.

As you clean up, breathe deeply and say thanks for the peace you just experienced. Now that you have reset your mind, your stress and anxiety will have less of a foothold.

Herbal tea is an excellent resource for boosting your immunity. You can create the perfect tea blend to achieve immune-boosting results to knock out the risk of illnesses. The final chapter will focus on using teas to boost your overall wellness.

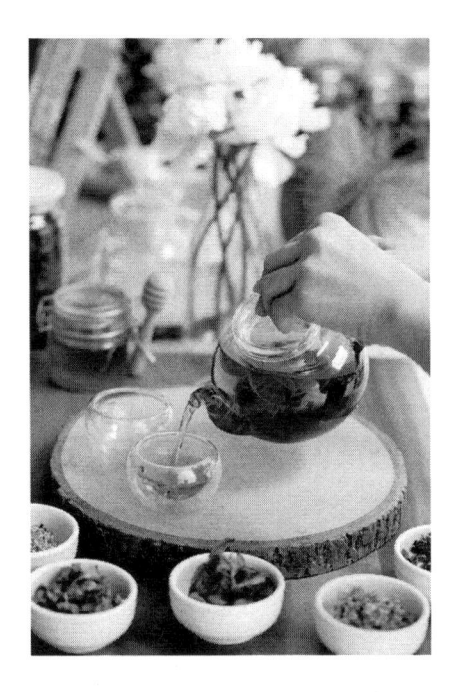

8

ACHIEVE SAGE SERENITY AND WELLNESS WITH THESE FINAL TEAS

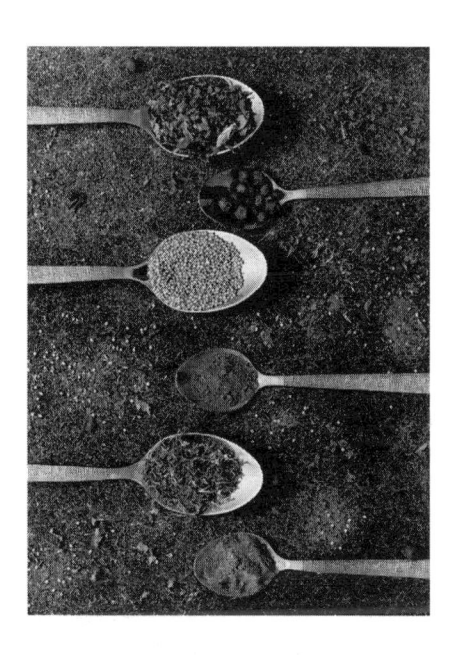

> *Tea is a part of daily life. It is as simple as eating when hungry and drinking when thirsty.*
>
> — YAMAMOTO SOSHUN

So far in our journey through the different types of teas, we've explored how they can help relieve stress and anxiety, induce good sleep, improve digestive health, and boost immunity. Many other teas can also benefit you by improving your overall wellness.

Robert consistently felt run down no matter what he did. One day, when he talked with his cousin Brad about how he felt, Brad suggested he try using wellness-enhancing teas. Deciding that it couldn't hurt to take his cousin's advice, Robert looked up a few tea recipes directed at some of his more pronounced symptoms. He ultimately found options that focused on a holistic path to wellness.

As he started drinking wellness-enhancing teas, Robert saw a marked difference in his overall health. Instead of feeling run down, he had more energy, increased focus, and a better outlook on life. From the effects of the tea, he felt inspired to incorporate more holistic practices that provided increasingly more benefits.

Like Robert, anyone can use wellness-enhancing teas to support their path to holistic wellness. It's important to understand that they are not a cure-all. Instead, they must be used in conjunction with a holistic lifestyle to achieve the most benefit.

We'll start by considering the path to holistic wellness to understand this.

THE PATH TO HOLISTIC WELLNESS

The concept of a healthy lifestyle varies from person to person. However, there are several similarities among all who lead healthy lives. They all practice the following healthy habits:

- eating a healthy diet
- participating in regular exercise
- maintaining a healthy body weight
- never smoking
- consuming alcohol in moderation if at all

When you practice a holistic lifestyle, you consider how all aspects of a healthy lifestyle come together to make you whole and well. Instead of focusing on just one part of a healthy lifestyle, you integrate all parts to consider yourself as a whole unit.

Many benefits come from leading a healthy lifestyle, some of which you may not even be aware of. Perhaps the most significant benefit you can receive is a longer lifespan. Let's say you've reached 50 years. If you combine all the healthy habits listed above, you could extend your life another 14 years. That said, implementing just a few of these changes now could significantly impact your longevity.

Embracing healthy habits can also significantly reduce your risk of developing various diseases, even if they run in your family. Following the rules of a healthy diet can help reduce the risk of cardiovascular disease and type 2 diabetes. Daily exercise at a moderate to vigorous intensity decreases the risk of death compared to those without exercise.

When you live a healthy lifestyle, you also simply feel better. As you slowly make and adapt to these changes, you'll move toward improved well-being. Making one change can lead you toward a cascade effect of many more positive changes, leading to even better overall feelings.

Knowing the habits of a healthy lifestyle is one thing. Knowing how to get there is another. These tips can be used as a guide to lead you down a holistic path toward a healthy lifestyle.

One of the first steps you can take is ensuring your diet is well-balanced. You should incorporate as many fruits and vegetables as possible when planning your meals. Additionally, they should be fresh whenever possible and never stored with high-sugar syrups. Strive for three servings of vegetables and two servings of fruits daily. Additionally, whenever you have refined grains, swap them for whole grains.

Adding more movement into your daily routine is also essential to a holistic approach to a healthy lifestyle. It's not just good for your physical health—it supports your mental health. Considering it more of moving your body than exercising may also help you get the task done, as many are put off by the concept of "working out." Choose an activity you enjoy that will keep you coming back for more. Start small and work your way toward a full session. Doing all these things will make you more likely to stick with it and improve your overall wellness.

Don't forget about getting enough sleep. Your body needs that time to recharge itself. When you don't get enough sleep, it can lead to decreased efficiency throughout your body and mind. You're less likely to make sound decisions, including good food choices, which will impact your overall health.

Hydration is also important. Whenever possible, choose clean, fresh water as your drink. Our bodies depend on water. Having enough ensures our brains and other organs operate at peak efficiency. If you're feeling parched or sluggish, a good drink of water may be just what you need.

Mental health is very important to your overall health and well-being. Maintaining friendships is a great way to boost your mental health and reduce your risk of depression. Isolation and poor relationships are closely linked to high risks of depression and several health problems, including headaches and pain (Risher, 2021).

When you have chronic stress, it can be very taxing on your immune system. In turn, you become more susceptible to health problems, including difficulty sleeping, cardiovascular problems, depression, and diabetes. You can combat stress through meditation, mindfulness, and exercise. If you're having difficulty on your own, don't be afraid to seek the help of a counselor.

Adding probiotics to your daily routine can also help reduce the risk of certain diseases. They're also great for boosting your gut health, which improves immunity. Consider ways to add them to your diet while they're fresh, like in fermented foods, to get the most impact.

When you shop, it's important to be mindful of certain toxins. Xenoestrogens include pesticides, bisphenol A (BPA), mycotoxins, polycyclic aromatic hydrocarbons (PAH), and so much more. Any of these can significantly damage your health. You'll need to be mindful that anything you buy doesn't contain these harmful toxins.

Ultimately, you must find something that motivates you to change your lifestyle. For example, focusing on being a smaller pants size will only work for so long before you either achieve that goal or become distracted. It needs to be something much more profound that keeps you going. Instead, focus on small goals that lead to big changes. Keeping too much focus on the big picture can lead to self-sabotage.

Instead of leaving certain things up to choice, put these healthy habits on automatic. Establish a basic menu that focuses on convenience. Make a schedule for your physical activity, striving to put something on daily. You can also track your food choices and activity with a handy app. There are tons to choose from that are free and easy to use.

You also need to care for your emotional health. When you have negative thoughts and emotions, you'll need to acknowledge them. However, don't let them stew. Instead, you should find ways to change how you respond to them and how you are thinking. Managing negative emotions can profoundly impact decreasing stress and promoting physical health.

A GUIDE TO WELLNESS-ENHANCING HERBS

Many herbs offer wellness-enhancing properties, ensuring you can get a significant boost when you add them to your diet. These are all excellent choices to work into a tea blend and can offer exceptional health benefits.

Cloves are often used in cooking, as they offer intense flavor notes. They've also been used in traditional medicine for centuries. They work to stimulate the circulatory system, promoting blood flow and warming the body. Additionally, cloves offer anti-inflammatory, analgesic, digestive, and antimicrobial properties.

Oregano is another common kitchen spice that also boosts overall wellness. It's rich in antioxidants and acts as a digestive aid and stimulant. Oregano can also support lung health while reducing inflammation.

Another kitchen herb, rosemary is great for mental health support. It can help improve your overall mood. It's an excellent choice for aiding in stress, anxiety, and depression relief.

Cinnamon has many uses due to having excellent antioxidant and antimicrobial properties. It is widely used to help reduce blood sugar levels. Additionally, some use it topically as a salve to reduce pain.

Turmeric is an excellent choice for its antioxidant properties. Its traditional uses have included protecting the heart, stabilizing blood sugar, protecting the heart, and reducing inflammation. Additionally, it's one of the main ingredients in a delicious curry recipe.

Thyme offers significant benefits above and beyond spicing your foods. It can help reduce blood pressure, fight infections, boost mood, and more.

Black peppercorns contain piperine, which is the source of their spicy kick. This compound may be able to help in the fight against some types of cancer. The science behind this is that piperine can trigger apoptosis, which is the mechanism that tells cells to self-destruct before they can grow out of control and develop tumors.

Cardamom is loaded with antioxidants, making it ideal for providing a wellness boost. It can help decrease blood pressure and may benefit those with gastrointestinal discomfort.

Cayenne pepper is spicy due to its capsaicin content. This component is ideal for boosting heart health. Additionally, it stimulates fat metabolism and aids in blood blotting.

Coriander is the cilantro plant's dried seeds. They contain the compound linalool, an antioxidant that may boast anti-cancer properties. Additionally, linalool may protect the brain from degenerative conditions and mood disorders.

Ginger has often been used to ease an upset stomach. However, it can do more than that. If you have a headache, it may be able to knock it out for you. It has analgesic properties, making it suitable for headaches, menstrual pain, and arthritis pain.

Paprika is another herb that contains capsaicin. This makes adding paprika to your foods or beverages ideal for reducing pain.

If you need an herb with a high antioxidant content, consider peppermint. It can be used to warm the body and stimulate circulation. It's also rich in vitamins and minerals. Many rely on it as a digestive aid, analgesic, and tension reliever. Additionally, it has antimicrobial properties.

The use of sage in the Middle Ages was strongly centered on preventing the plague. In more modern times, it's relied on to improve brain function and memory. Sage helps stop the breakdown of acetylcholine, which is a primary factor in the development of Alzheimer's disease.

Holy basil is different from traditional basil and Thai basil. It is considered to be sacred in India. It is an excellent option for reducing the growth of molds, yeasts, and bacteria. It can also boost immune system function by promoting specific immune cells in the bloodstream.

Originally used in Ayurvedic medicine for enhanced libido, fenugreek is now used for its beneficial effects on blood sugar. Daily consumption can improve the effects of the insulin hormone.

HEALTHY TEA RECIPES

Now that you have a basic idea of beneficial wellness-boosting herbs, it's time to put them to good use. Here are some excellent healthy tea recipes you can drink to holistically increase your overall health and wellness.

Pineapple Chamomile Basil Iced Tea

Sometimes, you just need to calm and center yourself before you start your day. This tea recipe can help you do that.

Ingredients:

- 1½ cups water
- 4 chamomile tea bags
- ½ cup frozen pineapple chunks
- honey to taste
- 2½ cups crushed ice
- 2 tbsp chopped basil

Directions:

1. Boil the water and remove from the heat.
2. Add the tea bags.
3. Steep for 2–3 minutes.
4. Allow the tea to cool
5. Combine the cooled tea, pineapple, honey, and 1 cup of ice in a blender.
6. Blend well.
7. Allow the contents to settle slightly, then stir in the basil.
8. Split the remaining ice between two glasses and add the tea to each glass.

To get the most flavor from this recipe, allow the tea to sit for as long as possible to have the different flavors mesh together (*Pineapple Chamomile Tea*, 2016).

Rosemary Orange Iced Tea

This tea offers bright flavors while offering antibacterial benefits from the rosemary.

Ingredients:

- 64 oz unsweetened iced tea
- 2 oranges
- 1 lemon
- 5 sprigs of rosemary

Directions:

1. Place the tea in a large pitcher.
2. Add the juice of one orange.
3. Slice the lemon and remaining orange. Place the slices in the pitcher.
4. Crush the rosemary with your hands, then add to the pitcher.
5. Let the tea sit for 4 hours at room temperature.
6. Strain and serve over ice. If desired, you can garnish it with orange slices and rosemary (Lisa, 2019).

Orange Mint Tea

This is an excellent choice if you're looking for a refreshing beverage that promotes overall wellness. It's perfect for a beautiful summer day.

Ingredients:

- 20 cups water
- 1 cup fresh mint
- 1 cup sugar
- 1 large navel orange
- 1–2 tbsp orange blossom water

Optional ingredients:

- orange slices
- additional mint

Directions:

1. Combine water and mint in a 6-quart slow cooker.
2. Cook on high for 6 hours.
3. Strain the mint and discard.
4. Add sugar and whisk until fully dissolved.
5. Halve the orange and squeeze the juice into the water.
6. Add orange blossom water.
7. Stir thoroughly to combine.
8. Transfer the tea to a pitcher.
9. Refrigerate for 4–6 hours or until cold.

10. Serve over ice and garnish with orange slices and additional mint as desired (*Orange Blossom Mint Refresher*, 2023).

Cucumber Mint Green Tea

Featuring the healing power of Japanese green tea, this recipe also packs a punch with the cooling powers of cucumber and mint.

Ingredients:

- 8 cups prepared Japanese green tea
- ¼ cup mint leaves, finely chopped and muddled
- ½ cup cucumber, peeled, seeded, and pureed
- ¼ cup freshly squeezed lime or lemon juice

Optional ingredients:

- fresh mint leaves
- cucumber slices
- simple syrup

Directions:

1. Combine tea, mint, cucumber puree, and lemon or lime juice in a large pitcher.
2. If desired, sweeten to taste.
3. Cover and chill for several hours.
4. If desired, strain before serving.

5. To serve, pour over ice and garnish with cucumber slices and mint leaves (Goodwin, 2022a).

Bella Basil Raspberry Tea

This recipe is full of the fresh taste of luscious raspberries and all the health benefits of basil, with a little fizzy kick you're sure to love.

Ingredients:

- ¼ cup lime juice
- 1 cup sugar
- 3 cups fresh raspberries
- 1 cup packed fresh basil leaves, coarsely chopped
- 2 black tea bags
- 32 oz carbonated water
- ice cubes

Directions:

1. Combine lime juice, sugar, raspberries, and basil in a large saucepan and mash the berries.
2. Cook over medium heat for approximately 7 minutes until the berries release their juices.
3. Remove the pan from the heat and add the tea bags.
4. Steep covered for 20 minutes.
5. Strain and transfer to a 2-quart pitcher.
6. Cover and refrigerate.

7. When you're ready to serve, slowly add the carbonated water.
8. Pour the tea over ice and garnish with additional fresh raspberries and basil (*Bella Basil Raspberry Tea*, 2023)l.

Lemon Basil Tea

You can enjoy a nice cup of tea flavored with lemon and basil. You'll also get a healthy boost to your overall health and wellness with each cup you drink.

Ingredients:

- 3 quarts water
- 1 cup fresh basil leaves, thinly sliced
- ¼ cup English breakfast tea leaves
- ¼ cup lemon zest, grated

Directions:

1. Boil water in a large saucepan.
2. Remove from the heat.
3. Add remaining ingredients.
4. Cover and steep for 4 minutes.
5. Strain and serve immediately (*Lemon Basil Tea*, 2023).

Hibiscus Iced Tea

This naturally sweet tea is calorie and caffeine free, offering a refreshing drink whenever needed.

Ingredients:

- 1 cup water
- 5 dried hibiscus flowers
- ice cubes

Directions:

1. Boil water and remove from the heat.
2. Add the flowers and steep for 5 minutes.
3. Strain and serve over ice (*Hibiscus Iced Tea*, 2022).

Green Tea With Grapefruit

Green tea, rosemary, and grapefruit combine to make this refreshing, healing tea.

Ingredients:

- 2 tsp green whole-leaf tea
- ¼ grapefruit, sliced
- sprig of rosemary
- honey or agave syrup to taste

Directions:

1. Add 5 ounces of cold water to a mug.
2. Top with 15 ounces of boiling water.
3. Add the tea leaves and steep for 2 minutes.

4. While the tea is steeping, add boiling water to a teapot to heat it.
5. Empty the teapot and place the grapefruit and rosemary inside.
6. Strain the green tea into the teapot.*
7. Allow this mixture to infuse for several minutes before serving.

*At this step, you can keep the tea leaves for a second brew later in the day. If you do this, the second time you steep the tea, do it for 3–4 minutes (Nice, n.d.-a).

Matcha With Vanilla

If you enjoy green tea, try this matcha blend. It's ready fast, so you don't have to wait.

Ingredients:

- seeds from ½ vanilla pod
- ½ tsp matcha powder

Directions:

1. Boil water in a kettle.
2. Pour 3 ounces into a measuring jug.
3. Pour half that water into a small bowl to heat it.
4. Add the ingredients to the remaining water in the measuring jug.

5. Whisk the mixture until completely smooth and slightly frothy.
6. Discard the water in the tea bowl and pour in the matcha blend (Nice, n.d.-b).

Anti-Inflammatory Weight-Loss Tea

This recipe is ideal for releasing excess water weight and bloat, providing a needed detox for your body.

Ingredients (use equal amounts of each):

- organic dried dandelion leaf
- organic dried willow bark
- dried hibiscus flowers
- dried ginger root
- high mallow

Directions:

1. Combine all ingredients and store them in a tightly sealed container.
2. To brew your tea, steep 1 tablespoon in 1 cup of boiling water for 3–5 minutes (Krystal, 2015).

Energy Herbal Tea

If you're looking for an all-natural pick-me-up, this tea offers exactly what you need.

Ingredients:

- ½ tsp loose green tea leaves
- 1 tsp rosemary
- ⅛ tsp nutmeg
- 8 oz boiling water
- honey, optional

Directions:

1. Add tea, rosemary, and nutmeg to an infuser.
2. Steep in the boiling water for 5–7 minutes.
3. Remove the infuser and sweeten it with honey if desired (Chef Mommie, n.d.).

Weight-Loss Green Tea

This low-calorie green tea can give you the boost you need to reach your weight-loss goals.

Ingredients:

- 1 tsp organic green tea leaves
- ½ cup fresh mint leaves
- ½ tsp organic honey

Directions:

1. Combine the tea leaves with 1 cup of boiling water.
2. Steep for several minutes, then strain the tea leaves out.

3. Wash, chop, and add the mint leaves to the cup.
4. Mix well.
5. Add honey to taste.
6. Serve warm or chilled (*Weight Loss*, 2022)

Brain Power-Up Tea

When you get that overwhelming feeling that slows you down in the afternoon, this tea will give you an excellent sustained pick-me-up.

Ingredients:

- lemongrass
- rosemary
- gotu kola
- turmeric
- tulsi

Directions:

1. Combine all ingredients in equal parts and store in a tightly sealed container.
2. To brew, steep 1 teaspoon in 1 cup of boiling water for 5–10 minutes.
3. Strain and enjoy (*3 Herbal Tea Recipes for Wellness*, n.d.)

M'Lady's Cup Tea

Chamomile and red raspberry leaf come together in this recipe to benefit the nervous system and digestive tract while alleviating inflammation.

Ingredients:

- ½ part peppermint or spearmint
- 1 part red raspberry leaf
- 1 part chamomile
- pinch of lavender

Directions:

1. Combine all ingredients and store them in a tightly sealed container.
2. To brew your tea, steep 1 teaspoon in 1 cup of boiling water until it reaches your desired strength (Atwood, 2017).

Love Tea

Enjoy this recipe yourself, or share it with friends and family as a lovely gift.

Ingredients:

- ¼ cup lavender blossoms
- ¾ cup jasmine blossoms
- ½ cup hibiscus flowers

- ¾ cup rose petals
- ½ cup rosemary

Directions:

1. Combine all ingredients and store them in a tightly sealed container.
2. To prepare your tea, steep 1 teaspoon per 1 cup of boiling water.
3. Steep for 10 minutes before drinking (Atwood, 2017).

Holy Basil Sage Tea

This tea recipe packs holy basil's medicinal power into each cup.

Ingredients:

- pinch of dried Sweet Annie leaves, optional
- ¼ cup dried holy basil leaves
- ¼ tsp dried powdered sage
- ½ tsp green tea

Directions:

1. Combine all ingredients and store them in a tightly sealed container.
2. To prepare your tea, steep 1 teaspoon per 1 cup of boiling water.
3. Steep for 10 minutes before drinking (Atwood, 2017).

Memory Tea

This tea can help your overall wellness in many ways, including aiding the female reproductive system, aiding asthma, and reducing inflammation.

Ingredients (use equal amounts of each):

- licorice root
- rosemary
- rose

Directions:

1. Combine all ingredients and store them in a tightly sealed container.
2. To brew your tea, steep 1 teaspoon in 1 cup of boiling water for 10 minutes (Atwood, 2017).

Garden Tea

Sage offers many benefits, including soothing sore throats and aiding digestion, making this a versatile tea.

Ingredients (use equal amounts of each):

- peppermint or spearmint
- purple sage leaves
- lemon balm
- rose petals

Directions:

1. Combine all ingredients and store them in a tightly sealed container.
2. To brew your tea, steep 1 teaspoon in 1 cup of boiling water for 10 minutes (Atwood, 2017).

Summer Sunshine Tea

Chamomile, peppermint, and sage come together in this recipe to stimulate health and wellness.

Ingredients:

- ¼ part lemon peel
- 1 part peppermint
- 1 part chamomile
- pinch of clove
- 1 part sage

Directions:

1. Combine all ingredients and store them in a tightly sealed container.
2. To brew your tea, steep 1 teaspoon in 1 cup of boiling water for 10 minutes (Atwood, 2017).

Sage Tea

This recipe is versatile and can be substituted with any type of sage you would like to use.

Ingredients:

- 4 cups water
- ¼ oz fresh sage leaves
- 1¼ tsp lemon zest
- 3 tbsp lemon juice
- 2 tbsp sugar

Directions:

1. Boil the water and reduce heat to a simmer.
2. Add the remaining ingredients, stirring well.
3. Steep for 20–30 minutes, stirring occasionally.
4. Strain.
5. Serve hot or over ice (Goodwin, 2022b).

INTERACTIVE ELEMENT

We've come to our last tea-drinking ritual together. As with the others before, we'll focus on relieving stress and anxiety as we prepare and enjoy our tea.

Whether you choose your tea for overall wellness or something else, let it be something that speaks to you in the moment. It should be something you will enjoy or else it will detract from the moment, causing displeasure that can add to your stress.

This time, choose a book of soothing words to accompany your tea. It can be poetry, supportive thoughts, or anything positive that resonates with you. As your water boils, listen to the changes in sounds coming from the kettle or pot. Be mindful of each action you take.

When you pour the water over your tea blend, pay close attention to how the color of the water changes and the leaves unfurl. As your tea steeps, begin reading the soothing words. Let them fill you and consume you. They should provide comfort in your time of need.

Pause your reading when the tea is ready. Take that first sip, savoring every action and flavor. Enjoy how it warms you from the top down. Continue reading as you finish the cup. When you are finished, take a moment to be grateful for the peace you just experienced.

Herbs offer us many ways to care for ourselves, promoting health and wellness in various forms. When used in tea blends, they make it enjoyable to approach a healthy lifestyle holistically. We've come to the end of our journey exploring herbal teas. In the final pages together, we'll wrap up with some final thoughts.

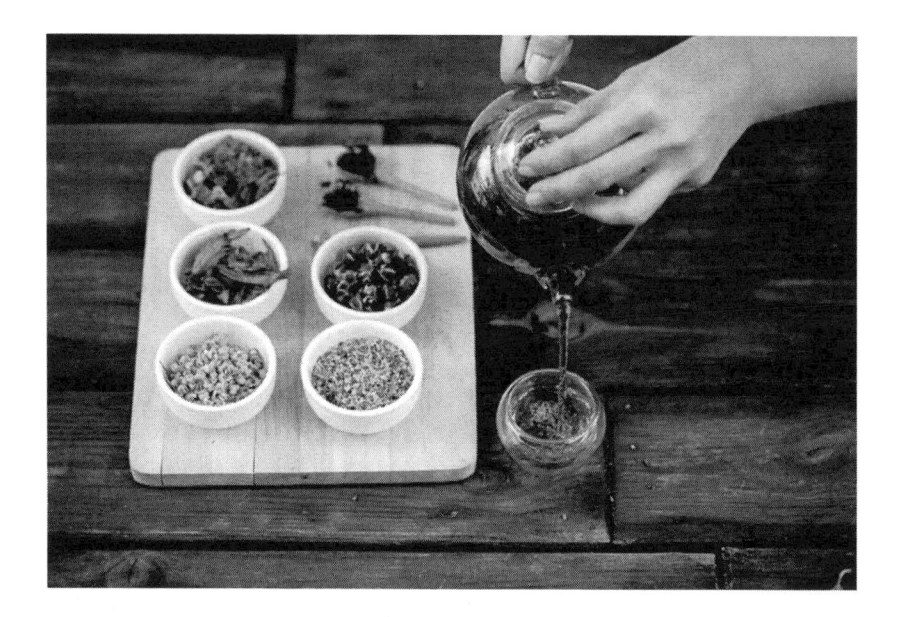

Good Health for All!

You're at the start of a transformative journey ... and what better time to light the path for someone else?

Simply by sharing your honest opinion of this book and a little about your own explorations with herbal teas, you'll help other people looking for natural health solutions to find the trustworthy guidance they're searching for.

LEAVE A REVIEW!

Thank you so much for your support. This is health advice we all deserve, and I'm grateful for your help in sharing it.

Scan the QR code to leave a review!

CONCLUSION

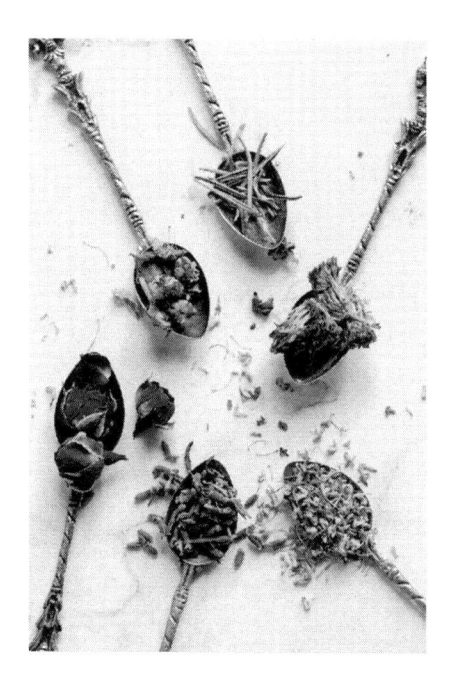

Herbal tea has a long, wonderful history of use that dates back to ancient times. From traditional medicine to tea-drinking ceremonies, it has a solid place in many cultures. Today, with more individuals seeking to be healthier, the focus on using herbal teas to achieve these goals is increasing.

We have explored the concept of TEAS:

- **T** - Tea's healing properties, fundamentals, and history
- **E** - Essential tips for taking a balanced and holistic approach to health and wellness
- **A** - Applicable safety tips for risk-free herbal tea drinking
- **S** - Scrumptious tea recipes

You now have the tools you need to prepare recipes for various aspects of health and wellness. Whether you need to break down the walls of stress and anxiety, get better sleep, improve digestion, increase immunity, or enhance your general wellness, you have many recipes to get you started on your journey.

While you may not be ready to give up on modern medicine like Heidi at the beginning of the book, you can take the steps she did to begin transforming your life. Focusing on what you put into your body can greatly affect how you feel daily. By adding herbal teas directed at your needs, you have the opportunity to enhance your overall health and well-being.

Throughout the pages of this book, we have seen the positive effects of herbal teas in all the personal stories. This is your opportunity to create your own story of success. Now that you know all the amazing powers and benefits of using herbal teas, all that's left for you to do is use them to your advantage and improve your life and health!

I would love to hear about your experiments with herbal teas. If you've enjoyed this book and had success with the recipes, please feel free to leave a review. This will help others looking for similar advice find exactly what they need.

Here's to a future of improved health and wellness!

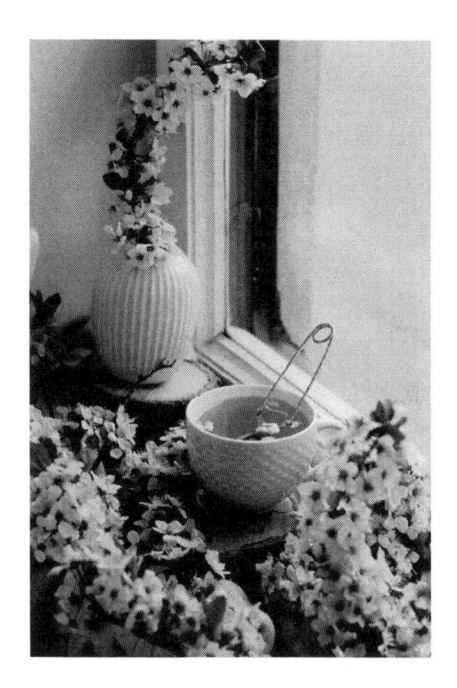

REFERENCES

"299+ Best Herbal Quotes For Inspiration [2024 Updated]." Grind Success. Last modified July 26, 2023. https://grindsuccess.com/herbal-quotes/

Aboelsoud, N. H. (2021, June 22). *Herbal medicine in ancient Egypt*. Brewminate. https://brewminate.com/herbal-medicine-in-ancient-egypt

Ackerman, C. E. (2017, March 6). *23 amazing health benefits of mindfulness for body and brain*. Positive Psychology. https://positivepsychology.com/benefits-of-mindfulness

Aivoges, E. (2023, January 9). *Herbal tea myths busted (Is it really safe to drink?)*. Kitchenicious. https://kitchenicious.com/are-herbal-teas-safe

Akhtar, A. (n.d.). *Easy homemade passion flower tea: How to dry and brew*. AtOnce. https://atonce.com/blog/how-to-dry-passion-flower-for-tea

Ali, S. (2021, June 15). *How to make a sparkling nightcap tea with herbs for better sleep*. Well+Good. https://www.wellandgood.com/herbs-for-sleep-tea-recipe

Anderson, E., & Zagorski, J. (2023, April 3). *Herbal tea*. Center for Research on Ingredient Safety. https://www.canr.msu.edu/news/herbal-tea

Anthis, C. (2014, September 18). *Ten homemade herbal teas for cold and flu season*. Herbal Academy. https://theherbalacademy.com/ten-homemade-herbal-teas-for-cold-and-flu-season

Asha. (2020, June 2). *Earl Grey and lavender iced tea*. Kitchen Fairy. https://kitchenfairy.co/blog/recipes/earl-grey-and-lavender-iced-tea/#tasty-recipes-4389-jump-target

Atwood, M. (2017, June 29). *20 essential herbal tea recipes: Tasty blends for health & comfort*. Selene River Press. https://www.seleneriverpress.com/20-essential-herbal-tea-recipes-tasty-blends-health-comfort

Azmanov, V. (2017, January 26). *Spiced ginger tea*. Veena Azmanov. https://veenaazmanov.com/5-spiced-ginger-tea-for-cold-and-sore-throat

Bedosky, L. (2022a, March 21). *5 types of tea that may support your immune system*. Everyday Health. https://www.everydayhealth.com/diet-nutrition/types-of-tea-that-may-help-support-your-immune-system

Bedosky, L. (2022b, December 1). *7 herbs and spices that may help boost immu-*

nity naturally. Everyday Health. https://www.everydayhealth.com/diet-nutrition/herbs-and-spices-that-may-help-boost-immunity-naturally

Bella basil raspberry tea. (2023, September 12). Taste of Home. https://www.tasteofhome.com/recipes/bella-basil-raspberry-tea

The benefits of holistic approaches to health and wellness. (n.d.). Operation Red Wings Foundation. https://orwfoundation.org/the-benefits-of-holistic-approaches-to-health-and-wellness

Berardi, R. (2021, July 26). *Origin and history of herbal tea: The benefits for body and mind*. FV Magazine. https://magazine.fortevillageresort.com/wellness/origin-and-history-of-herbal-tea-the-benefits-for-body-and-mind/?lang=en

Bibe. (2020, April 21). *Which teas are good for improving digestion?* My Folk Medicine. https://www.myfolkmedicine.com/which-teas-are-good-for-improving-digestion

Blackwood, M. (2021, November 5). *Immunity booster tea*. Healthier Steps. https://healthiersteps.com/recipe/immunity-booster-tea

Blankespoor, J. (2013, June 4). *Herbal infusions and decoctions: Preparing medicinal teas*. Chestnut School of Herbal Medicine. https://chestnutherbs.com/herbal-infusions-and-decoctions-preparing-medicinal-teas

Bous, S., & Neveln, V. (2023, July 5). *5 methods for how to dry herbs for cooking and crafting*. Better Homes & Gardens. https://www.bhg.com/gardening/vegetable/herbs/drying-herbs

Breo Box. (2023, October 11). *Tea time rituals: Creating a relaxing tea-sipping experience*. Breo Box Blog. https://www.breobox.com/blogs/news/tea-time-rituals

Bryant Shrader, M. (2021, April 10). *How to make a great night's sleep herb tea*. Mary's Nest. https://marysnest.com/how-to-make-a-great-nights-sleep-herb-tea

Camila. (2022, December 9). *Best herbal tea recipes for anxiety and calming stress*. Brewed Leaf Love. https://brewedleaflove.com/herbal-tea-stress-anxiety

Caplan, E. (2021, July 28). *The 13 best herbal teas for stress relief, brain health, and more*. Healthline. https://www.healthline.com/health/mental-health/tea-for-stress

Carrie. (2021, January 21). *10 soothing tea recipes for colds, coughs, and flu*. Brewed Leaf Love. https://brewedleaflove.com/tea-recipes-for-colds

Carrie. (2022, July 23). *How to make copycat Starbucks Medicine Ball Tea recipe*. Brewed Leaf Love. https://brewedleaflove.com/starbucks-medicine-ball

Carrie, A. (2020, November 23). *Tea time traditions around the world.* Brewed Leaf Love. https://brewedleaflove.com/tea-time-traditions

Cartwright, M. (2017, July 10). *Tea in Ancient China & Japan.* World History Encyclopedia. https://www.worldhistory.org/article/1093/tea-in-ancient-china--japan

Chef Mommie. (n.d.). *Energy Herbal Tea Recipe.* Food. https://www.food.com/recipe/energy-herbal-tea-186759

Cherry, K. (2022, September 2). *Benefits of mindfulness.* Verywell Mind. https://www.verywellmind.com/the-benefits-of-mindfulness-5205137

Choe, J. (2018, January 24). *Easy chamomile tea latte.* Oh, How Civilized. https://www.ohhowcivilized.com/chamomile-tea-latte/?utm_content=buffer27032&utm_medium=social&utm_source=pinterest.com&utm_campaign=buffer

Christodoulou, M. (2019, August 25). *Medicinal herbs in ancient Greece.* The Greek Herbalist. https://www.thegreekherbalist.com/herbalcolumn/medicinalherbsinancientgreece

Coelho, S. (2022, June 23). *The 20 best teas for anxiety.* Healthline. https://www.healthline.com/health/anxiety/tea-for-anxiety

Coetzee, M. (2019, March 13). *What is Cha-Dao? Learn how to hold a simple tea ceremony.* WellBeing Magazine. https://www.wellbeing.com.au/body/health/cha-dao-tea-drink-drinking-chinense.html

Cohen, S. (2020, March 16). *How to make an herbal immune tea.* Suzy Cohen. https://suzycohen.com/articles/how-to-make-an-herbal-immune-tea

Complete guide to herbal tea. (n.d.). Full Leaf Tea Company. https://fullleafteacompany.com/pages/what-is-herbal-tea

Cooks-Campbell, A. (2021, August 12). *Holistic wellness is a real thing. Here's why you need it.* BetterUp. https://www.betterup.com/blog/holistic-wellness

Covington, L. (2023, August 24). *How to dry herbs: 4 simple ways.* The Spruce Eats. https://www.thespruceeats.com/harvesting-and-drying-leafy-herbs-1327541

Daniel. (2021, August 7). *Can you drink too much herbal tea? (And what happens?).* Let's Drink Tea! https://letsdrinktea.com/can-you-drink-too-much-herbal-tea

Daniela. (2018, June 26). *DIY sleep time herbal tea.* Tea Cachai. https://www.teacachai.com/diy-night-time-herbal-tea

Davis, T. (2020, December 7). *6 easy steps to a healthier lifestyle.* Psychology

Today. https://www.psychologytoday.com/us/blog/click-here-happiness/202012/6-easy-steps-healthier-lifestyle

de la Forêt, R. (2016, December 8). *Tea blend recipes for gift giving*. LearningHerbs. https://learningherbs.com/remedies-recipes/tea-blend-recipes-2

Debi. (2015, April 14). *Cinnamon sore throat tea*. Life Currents. https://lifecurrentsblog.com/cinnamon-sore-throat-tea

Dessinger, H. (2015, May 15). *Sweet dreams tea recipe*. Mommypotamus. https://mommypotamus.com/sweet-dreams-tea/

Dix, M., & Klein, E. (2018, July 2). *Understanding gut health: Signs of an unhealthy gut and what to do about it*. Healthline. https://www.healthline.com/health/gut-health#_noHeaderPrefixedContent

Downs, A. (2023, October 2). *All the tea (not) in China: The story of how India became a tea-drinking nation*. Serious Eats. https://www.seriouseats.com/indian-tea-history-5221096

EatingWell Test Kitchen. (n.d.). *Warm honey green tea*. EatingWell. https://www.eatingwell.com/recipe/266309/warm-honey-green-tea

EatingWell Test Kitchen. (2023, September 19). *Soothing ginger-lemon tea*. EatingWell. https://www.eatingwell.com/recipe/259696/soothing-ginger-lemon-tea

Edgar, J. (2009, March 20). *Types of teas and their health benefits*. WebMD. https://www.webmd.com/diet/features/tea-types-and-their-health-benefits

8 simple, homemade herbal tea recipes. (2020, March 17). Simple Loose Leaf Tea Company. https://simplelooseleaf.com/blog/herbal-tea/herbal-tea-recipes

11 herbs you need to know for immune support. (2022, April 4). Gaia Herbs. https://www.gaiaherbs.com/blogs/seeds-of-knowledge/11-herbs-you-need-to-know-for-immune-support

Enhancing well-being: The power of rituals and the art of drinking tea. (2023, July 25). Bredemeijer. https://www.bredemeijer.com/blog/enhancing-well-being-the-power-of-rituals-and-the-art-of-drinking-tea

Fanous, S. (2014, November 4). *12 health benefits of thyme*. Healthline. https://www.healthline.com/health/health-benefits-of-thyme

Ferko, T. (2020, March 20). *Homemade ginger & lemon tea with turmeric*. My Vegan Minimalist. https://myveganminimalist.com/ayurvedic-ginger-turmeric-tea

REFERENCES | 203

Foods4Health. (n.d.). *Drink clove and cinnamon tea each morning, this will happen to your body!* YouTube. https://www.youtube.com/watch?v=LxCtLXu6VsI&t=2s

Gardenuity. (2019, December 31). *Fresh herbal teas | the ultimate guide*. The Sage. https://blog.gardenuity.com/fresh-herbal-teas-the-ultimate-guide

Goodwin, L. (2022a, May 24). *Cucumber mint green iced tea*. The Spruce Eats. https://www.thespruceeats.com/cucumber-mint-green-tea-recipe-765431

Goodwin, L. (2022b, December 8). *Sage herbal tea recipe*. The Spruce Eats. https://www.thespruceeats.com/sage-tea-recipe-766393

Groves, M. N. (2019, March 27). *Herbs for digestion (plus a gut-healing tea blend)*. LearningHerbs. https://learningherbs.com/remedies-recipes/gut-healing-tea

Halliwell, E. (2016, November 16). *How to be mindful with a cup of tea*. Mindful. https://www.mindful.org/mindful-cup-tea/

Han, E. (2020, January 29). *Recipe: after-dinner belly-soothing tea*. Kitchn. https://www.thekitchn.com/recipe-afterdinner-bellysoothing-tea-recipes-from-the-kitchn-200050

Harper. (2023, July 18). *Where to find affordable herbal tea*. Sally Tea Cups. https://sallyteacups.org/where-to-find-affordable-herbal-tea

Harvard Health. (2019, March 21). *Benefits of mindfulness*. Help Guide. https://www.helpguide.org/harvard/benefits-of-mindfulness.htm

Hawthorne, S. (2016, December 12). *A simple guide to digestive wellness*. Food Matters. https://www.foodmatters.com/article/a-simple-guide-to-digestive-wellness

Hayes, A. (n.d.). *How to create your own (tea time) rituals*. Plum Deluxe Tea. https://www.plumdeluxe.com/blogs/blog/how-to-create-your-own-tea-time-rituals

Healey, J. (2017, December 19). *5 stress relief tea blends to make your day better*. Healing Brave. https://healingbrave.com/blogs/all/stress-relief-tea-blends

The health benefits of 3 herbal teas. (2021, October 21). Harvard Health. https://www.health.harvard.edu/nutrition/the-health-benefits-of-3-herbal-teas

Healthline Editorial Team. (2020, February 25). *Everything you need to know about stress*. Healthline. https://www.healthline.com/health/stress

Healthy tea recipes. (n.d.). BBC Good Food. https://www.bbcgoodfood.com/recipes/collection/healthy-tea-recipes

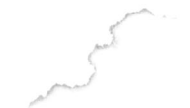

Heidi. (2022, November 21). *Best herbs for digestion + 3 easy recipes*. Mountain Rose Herbs. https://blog.mountainroseherbs.com/herbs-healthy-digestion-recipes

Helmy Abou El-Soud, N. (2010). Herbal medicine in ancient Egypt. *Journal of Medicinal Plants Research, 4*(2), 82–86. https://www.researchgate.net/publication/228634623_Herbal_medicine_in_ancient_Egypt

Herbal sleep tea – the ultimate, effective and easy, recipe. (2014, September 14). Little Homesteaders. https://littlehomesteaders.com/herbal-sleep-tea-ultimate-effective-easy-recipe/#google_vignette

Herbal tea recipe for sleep. (2013, April 24). The Elliott Homestead. https://theelliotthomestead.com/2013/04/cinnamon-sleep-tonic

Herman, E. (2020, March 30). *Enjoy an immune system boost: 4 recipes for your own herbal tea*. Art of Living. https://www.artofliving.org/us-en/blog/enjoy-an-immune-system-boost-4-recipes-for-your-own-herbal-tea

Hibiscus iced tea. (2022, October 5). Taste of Home. https://www.tasteofhome.com/recipes/hibiscus-iced-tea

The hidden health benefits of tea. (2019, December 9). Penn Medicine. https://www.pennmedicine.org/updates/blogs/health-and-wellness/2019/december/health-benefits-of-tea

Hill, A. (2023, March 24). *9 side effects of drinking too much tea*. Healthline. https://www.healthline.com/nutrition/side-effects-of-tea

The history of herbal tea. (n.d.). Revolution Tea. https://www.revolutiontea.com/blogs/news/the-history-of-herbal-tea

History of herbal tea. (2021, October 5). Journey Leaf. https://journeyleaftea.com/blogs/news/history-of-herbal-tea

Hoffmaster, D. (2023, June 22). *How to make your own herbal teas*. Treehugger. https://www.treehugger.com/how-to-make-your-own-herbal-tea-recipes-and-instructions-5194393

Holistic wellness: What is it and why is it important? (2022, January 6). Goalcast. https://www.goalcast.com/holistic-wellness

Homemade dried fruit and herb tea. (n.d.). Whole Foods Market. https://www.wholefoodsmarket.com/recipes/homemade-dried-fruit-and-herb-tea

How important the tea was in Ancient China? (2023, November 1). China Culture. http://en.chinaculture.org/focus/2013-06/04/content_461822.htm

How much sleep is enough? (2022, March 24). NIH. https://www.nhlbi.nih.gov/health/sleep/how-much-sleep

How to boost your immune system. (2021, February 15). Harvard Health. https://www.health.harvard.edu/staying-healthy/how-to-boost-your-immune-system

How to hold a tea ceremony as an act of self-care. (2022, March 2). Cedar and Myrrh. https://cedarandmyrrh.com/blogs/news/how-to-hold-a-tea-ceremony-as-an-act-of-self-care

How to make sleepy time tea. (n.d.). Crane & Canopy. https://www.craneandcanopy.com/pages/how-to-make-sleepy-time-tea

How to make your own homemade herbal tea. (n.d.). Brod & Taylor. https://brodandtaylor.com/blogs/recipes/how-to-make-your-own-tea-blends

How to talk to your doctor or health care provider. (n.d.). Student Health and Wellness Services. https://health.williams.edu/medical-diagnoses/general-health-concerns/how-to-talk-to-your-doctor-or-health-care-provider

Howley, E. K. (2018, January 16). *How to make sure your doctor understands your medical condition.* U.S. News and World Report. https://health.usnews.com/health-care/patient-advice/articles/2018-01-16/how-to-make-sure-your-doctor-understands-your-medical-condition

Hu, S. (2020, March 22). *Immune-boosting ginger turmeric tea.* Ahead of Thyme. https://www.aheadofthyme.com/immune-boosting-ginger-turmeric-tea

James, M. (2013, October 8). *Herbs for digestion.* Women's Health Network. https://www.womenshealthnetwork.com/digestive-health/herbal-remedies-for-digestive-system

Jamie. (2014, July 10). *How to get your best sleep ever with calming tea.* The Herbal Spoon. https://www.theherbalspoon.com/sweet-sleep-tea

Jaswal, J. (2021, August 2). *6 best herbal teas to boost immune system.* HealthKart. https://www.healthkart.com/connect/6-best-herbal-tea-to-boost-immune-system

Jeanroy, A. (2022, August 12). *How to make your own herb tea blends.* The Spruce Eats. https://www.thespruceeats.com/make-your-own-herb-tea-blend-1762127

Jennings, K.-A., & Mathis, A. (2023, July 18). *14 of the world's healthiest spices & herbs you should be eating.* EatingWell. https://www.eatingwell.com/article/32764/eight-of-the-worlds-healthiest-spices-herbs-you-should-be-eating

Johnson, A. (2019, January 29). *Lemon ginger tea.* She Wears Many Hats. https://shewearsmanyhats.com/lemon-ginger-tea-recipe

Jones, E. (2023, September 28). *The mindful way to enjoy tea.* Juicer Advices. https://juiceradvices.com/mindfulness-and-tea-culture

Kampo: Traditional Japanese herbal medicine - an introduction. (2019, March 6). Iyashi Herbs. https://www.iyashiherbs.com/post/kampo-traditional-japanese-herbal-medicine-an-introduction

Karen, S. (2020, May 29). *Calming tea recipe & natural stress management (with video!).* Herbal Academy. https://theherbalacademy.com/calming-tea-recipe

Katja. (2017, September 26). *Best homemade tea blends for stress.* Wild for Nature. https://www.wildfornature.com/simple-guide-best-homemade-herbal-tea-blends-stress-anxiety

Keegan, K. (2015, December 31). *Mom lost 106 pounds in one year drinking weight-loss tea.* Redbook. https://www.redbookmag.com/body/health-fitness/news/a39094/woman-drops-106-pounds-green-tea-secret-weight-loss-success

Kelly. (2020, October 15). *The best herbal cold remedy tea recipe.* Montana Happy. https://montanahappy.com/cold-remedy-tea

Kelly. (2021, February 26). *Best herbal bedtime tea * sleep tea recipe.* Montana Happy. https://montanahappy.com/bedtime-tea-recipe

Kelly, K. (2020, December 16). *My tea ritual was a source of comfort during a terrible 2020.* Teen Vogue. https://www.teenvogue.com/story/tea-ritual-soothing-pandemic

Kiyomi. (2021, September 28). *Tea ritual guide.* Sei Mee Tea LLC. https://groundgreentea.com/blog/tea-ritual-guide

Kloss, K. (2023, June 21). *Can certain types of tea really help you sleep?* Livestrong. https://www.livestrong.com/article/13732096-best-tea-for-sleep

Krystal. (2015, March 24). *Anti-inflammatory weight loss tea.* Dishing up Balance. https://dishingupbalance.com/anti-inflammatory-weight-loss-tea

Lamoreaux, K. (2022, March 9). *The 10 best teas for stress in 2022.* Psych Central. https://psychcentral.com/health/tea-for-stress

Laurence, E. (2020, July 29). *7 healthy iced tea recipes that lower inflammation while quenching your thirst.* Well+Good. https://www.wellandgood.com/healthy-iced-tea-recipes

Lederle, D. (2019, July 29). *Stress relief tea.* The Healthy Maven. https://www.thehealthymaven.com/diy-stress-relief-tea

Leech, J. (2017, June 4). *10 delicious herbs and spices with powerful health benefits.* Healthline. https://www.healthline.com/nutrition/10-healthy-herbs-and-spices#TOC_TITLE_HDR_2

Lemon and ginger calming tonic. (n.d.). The Better Nutrition Program. https://thebetternutritionprogram.com/recipes/lemon-ginger-calming-tonic

Lemon basil tea. (2023, June 27). Taste of Home. https://www.tasteofhome.com/recipes/lemon-basil-tea

Levine, H. (2020, May 5). *5 ways to boost your immune system.* AARP. https://www.aarp.org/health/healthy-living/info-2020/boosting-immune-response.html

Li, C., Wu, F., Yuan, W., Ding, Q., Wang, M., Zhang, Q., Zhang, J., Xing, J., & Wang, S. (2019). Systematic review of herbal tea (a traditional Chinese treatment method) in the therapy of chronic simple pharyngitis and preliminary exploration about its medication rules. *Evidence-Based Complementary and Alternative Medicine, 2019,* 1–15. https://doi.org/10.1155/2019/9458676

Lilly, C. (2023, February 21). *Best digestive tea recipe.* Good Food Baddie. https://goodfoodbaddie.com/best-digestive-tea-recipe

Lisa. (2019, May 23). *Rosemary orange ice tea.* Lisa's Dinnertime Dish. https://lisasdinnertimedish.com/rosemary-orange-ice-tea

Loewe, E. (2022, January 19). *The best teas for dress relief & how to brew your perfect cup.* Mindbodygreen. https://www.mindbodygreen.com/articles/teas-for-stress

Loh, A. (2020, November 25). *11 soothing tea recipes for a relaxing night.* EatingWell. https://www.eatingwell.com/gallery/7874677/hot-tea-recipes

Lucy. (2022, October 14). *Sleep tea recipe (with banana peel).* LB Health & Lifestyle. https://lbhealthandlifestyle.com/sleep-tea-recipe-ease-anxiety-stress-insomnia

Manaker, L. (2023, March 20). *The benefits of drinking herbal teas for relaxation and health.* Verywell Health. https://www.verywellhealth.com/herbal-tea-health-and-anxiety-benefits-7255523

Mandriota, M. (2022, March 9). *All about the cycle of anxiety: What it is and how to cope.* Psych Central. https://psychcentral.com/anxiety/cycle-of-anxiety

Manteiga, R., Park, D. L., & Ali, S. S. (1997). Risks associated with consumption of herbal teas. *Reviews of Environmental Contamination and Toxicology, 150,* 1–30. https://doi.org/10.1007/978-1-4612-2278-1_1

Martha Stewart Test Kitchen. (2019, January 22). *Good-digestion tea.* Martha Stewart. https://www.marthastewart.com/1155941/good-digestion-tea

McGruther, J. (2021, December 9). *Sleepy tea.* Nourished Kitchen. https://nourishedkitchen.com/sleepy-tea-recipe

Mendicino, S. (2023, April 5). *6 herbs high in antioxidants*. The Botanical Institute. https://botanicalinstitute.org/herbs-high-in-antioxidants

Meredith, D. (2023, June 15). *31 tea recipes you haven't made yet*. Taste of Home. https://www.tasteofhome.com/collection/tea-recipes-you-havent-made-yet

Mike. (2018, February 1). *Tea mindfulness: Meditation and self-awareness in a cup*. The Tea Letter. https://thetealetter.com/tea-and-mindfulness/tea-mindfulness-meditation-making-tea

Modern African Table. (n.d.). *Easy cardamom ginger chai*. YouTube. https://www.youtube.com/watch?v=SaJZAAc5SqY

Mollenkamp, A. (2015, February 1). *Ginger mint green iced tea recipe*. Salt & Wind Travel. https://saltandwind.com/ginger-mint-green-iced-tea-recipe

Momaya, A. (2020, March 26). *Top 9 home-made drinks to strengthen your immune system*. HealthifyMe Blog. https://www.healthifyme.com/blog/top-9-home-made-drinks-to-strengthen-your-immune-system

Mulumba, P. (2020, May 3). *12 teas to boost your immune system*. Longevity. https://longevitylive.com/anti-aging/12-teas-boost-immune-system

Murphy, J. (2018, December 26). *This Napa Valley vintner's ritual for inner calm is a meditation*. Yoga Journal. https://www.yogajournal.com/meditation/ritual-for-inner-calm-is-better-than-meditation/

naturalherballiving. (2022, August 20). *Herbal tea recipes - healthy homemade teas from herbs*. Natural Herbal Living. https://naturalherballiving.com/herbal-tea-recipes

Nectar Sleep Editorial Team. (2021, June 28). *Herbs for sleep - 13 best herbs to improve your sleep*. Nectar Sleep. https://www.nectarsleep.com/posts/herbs-for-sleep

Nice, M. (n.d.-a). *Green tea with grapefruit*. BBC Good Food. https://www.bbcgoodfood.com/recipes/green-tea-grapefruit

Nice, M. (n.d.-b). *Matcha with vanilla*. BBC Good Food. https://www.bbcgoodfood.com/recipes/matcha-vanilla

Orange blossom mint refresher. (2023, September 12). Taste of Home. https://www.tasteofhome.com/recipes/orange-blossom-mint-refresher

Osiadacz, A. (2022, February 17). *Mayo Clinic minute: How to maintain a healthy immune system*. Mayo Clinic News Network. https://newsnetwork.mayoclinic.org/discussion/mayo-clinic-minute-how-to-maintain-a-healthy-immune-system/

Osmun, R. (2020). *12 natural herbs for sleep*. Eachnight. https://eachnight.com/sleep/12-natural-herbs-for-sleep

Paleohacks. (2016, February 29). *The ultimate 2-ingredient tea to drink when you're stressed*. Thrive Market. https://thrivemarket.com/blog/the-ultimate-2-ingredient-tea-to-drink-when-youre-stressed

Panchal, B. (2019, November 1). *What's the best tea for sleep? 7 recipes to try tonight*. Lifehack. https://www.lifehack.org/851858/best-tea-for-sleep

Pannunzio, L. A. (2020, March 31). *Tea meditation for beginners*. The Cup of Life. https://theteacupoflife.com/2020/03/tea-meditation-for-beginners.html

Pannunzio, L. A. (2023, August 10). *38 tea quotes that will inspire every tea drinker*. The Cup of Life. https://theteacupoflife.com/2020/07/tea-quotes.html

Perry, L. (2021, March 30). *Easy homemade tea for digestion*. Darn Good Veggies. https://www.darngoodveggies.com/easy-homemade-tea-for-digestion

Piccolo, M. (2019, December 1). *Drying herbs in the oven: Everything you need to know*. Drying All Foods. https://dryingallfoods.com/drying-herbs-in-the-oven

Pineapple chamomile tea. (2016, January 5). Chocolate for Basil. https://www.chocolateforbasil.com/blog/pineapple-chamomile-tea?rq=iced%20tea

Pittman, V. (2017, December 7). *Ancient medicine, herbs and herbal practice*. Herbal History Research Network. https://www.herbalhistory.org/home/ancient-medicine-herbs-and-herbal-practice

Power of Positivity. (2021, May 5). *How to make stress relief tea 4 ways*. Power of Positivity: Positive Thinking & Attitude. https://www.powerofpositivity.com/stress-relief-teas-4-easy-recipes

Powers, D. (2022, February 27). *The 11 best herbs for sleep & insomnia*. The Botanical Institute. https://botanicalinstitute.org/best-herbs-for-sleep

Powers, D. (2023, September 26). *The 5 best online herb suppliers | the complete buying guide*. The Botanical Institute. https://botanicalinstitute.org/best-herb-suppliers

Puchko, K. (2016, January 2). *15 tea traditions from around the world*. Mental Floss. https://www.mentalfloss.com/article/72891/15-tea-traditions-around-world

Purkh Singh Khalsa, K. (2020, December 28). *30 digestive herbs*. Mother Earth

Living. https://www.motherearthliving.com/health-and-wellness/digestive-herbs-zm0z12amzdeb

Resler, H. (2016, April 16). *43 tea recipes to instantly de-stress*. Paleo Blog. https://blog.paleohacks.com/tea-recipes

Richards, L. (2020, October 27). *3-day gut reset: Does it work?* Medical News Today. https://www.medicalnewstoday.com/articles/3-day-gut-reset

Rick. (2023, January 6). *Lemon mint iced tea recipe*. Paleo Leap. https://paleoleap.com/lemon-mint-iced-tea

Risher, B. (2021, January 6). *Healthy lifestyle benefits: 5 tips for living your strongest, healthiest life yet*. Healthline. https://www.healthline.com/health/fitness-nutrition/healthy-lifestyle-benefits

Ritual relaxation: How to host a healing tea ceremony. (n.d.). Sips By. https://www.sipsby.com/blogs/news/how-to-host-a-healing-tea-ceremony

Robertson, L. (2018, March 20). *20 beneficial herbal tea recipes that will comfort your body*. Morning Chores. https://morningchores.com/herbal-tea-recipes

Ros Walford. (2017, May 15). *A rough guide to: The Japanese tea ceremony*. Rough Guides. https://www.roughguides.com/article/a-rough-guide-to-the-japanese-tea-ceremony

Rose, A. (n.d.). *Poppy tea (yes, poppy!) for insomnia, anxiety, and nervousness!* Fresh Bites Daily. https://freshbitesdaily.com/poppy-tea

Saba, H. (2019, September 18). *How to formulate a gut-nourishing herbal tea blend*. Herbal Academy. https://theherbalacademy.com/gut-nourishing-herbal-tea-blend

Sarah. (2020, December 1). *10 warm and comforting herbal tea recipes to improve your sleep naturally*. Sarah Blooms. https://sarahblooms.com/herbal-tea-recipes

Schumer, L. (2023, April 21). *13 tea recipes you can easily brew up at home*. The Spruce Eats. https://www.thespruceeats.com/best-tea-recipes-4801911

The science of sleep: Understanding what happens when you sleep. (2019). Johns Hopkins Medicine Health Library. https://www.hopkinsmedicine.org/health/wellness-and-prevention/the-science-of-sleep-understanding-what-happens-when-you-sleep

Scott, E. (2022, November 7). *What is stress?* Verywell Mind. https://www.verywellmind.com/stress-and-health-3145086

Sherman, E. (2020, May 28). *How to conduct your own traditional Japanese tea ceremony*. Matador Network. https://matadornetwork.com/read/conduct-traditional-japanese-tea-ceremony

Six tips to enhance immunity. (2022, January 21). Centers for Disease Control and Prevention. https://www.cdc.gov/nccdphp/dnpao/features/enhance-immunity/index.html

Stanley, K. M. (2012, August 27). *Jack Frost tea*. Nourishing Simplicity. https://nourishingsimplicity.org/jack-frost-tea

Stormy. (2023, April 8). *How to source high-quality, organic herbs without breaking the bank*. The Happy Herbal Home. https://thehappyherbalhome.com/find-high-quality-herbs

Strengthen your immune system with 4 simple strategies. (2020, April 13). Health Essentials from Cleveland Clinic. https://health.clevelandclinic.org/strengthen-your-immune-system-with-simple-strategies

Suni, E. (2020a, October 23). *How sleep works: Understanding the science of sleep*. Sleep Foundation. https://www.sleepfoundation.org/how-sleep-works

Suni, E. (2020b, October 30). *What happens when you sleep*. Sleep Foundation. https://www.sleepfoundation.org/how-sleep-works/what-happens-when-you-sleep

Superfoodly. (2020, February 18). *How to make magnolia bark tea for sleep & anxiety*. Superfoodly. https://superfoodly.com/magnolia-bark-tea

Susannah. (2020, December 3). *20 calming herbs for relaxation & stress relief*. HealthyGreenSavvy. https://www.healthygreensavvy.com/calming-herbs-relaxation-stress

Susannah. (2022, January 10). *How to make lemon balm tea from fresh or dried lemon balm {3 delicious medicinal recipes}*. HealthyGreenSavvy. https://www.healthygreensavvy.com/how-to-make-lemon-balm-tea-recipe

Sutton, J. (2019, June 19). *20+ health benefits of meditation according to science*. Positive Psychology. https://positivepsychology.com/benefits-of-meditation

Sweetser, R. (2023, July 5). *Drying your own herbs for tea*. Old Farmer's Almanac. https://www.almanac.com/drying-your-own-herbs-tea

Szaro, M. (2022, May 27). *How to make your own tea blends + a soothing sleep tea recipe*. Herbal Academy. https://theherbalacademy.com/tea-blends

Tahmaseb-McConatha, J. (2022, July 6). *Taking time for tea: Comforting rituals in stressful times*. Psychology Today. https://www.psychologytoday.com/us/blog/live-long-and-prosper/202207/taking-time-tea-comforting-rituals-in-stressful-times

Tea drinking - A different gateway to spirituality. (2022, April 13). MindfulSouls. https://mindfulsouls.com/blogs/spirituality/tea-drinking-a-different-gateway-to-spirituality

Tea for meditation: A complete guide. (2023, July 4). Relax like a Boss. https://relaxlikeaboss.com/tea-for-meditation

Tea meditation - how to find calm with a cup of tea. (n.d.). Gabriela Green. https://gabriela.green/tea-meditation

Tea: A cup of good health? (2014, August 13). Harvard Health. https://www.health.harvard.edu/staying-healthy/tea-a-cup-of-good-health

Tea's rituals for your wellbeing: Sip, savor, and relax. (2023, August 2). Black Scottie Chai. https://blackscottiechai.com/sip-savor-and-relax-teas-rituals-for-your-wellbeing

Teajoy Editorial Team. (2023, July 19). *Brewing health and wellness: How to make ginseng tea*. TeaJoy. https://www.teajoy.com/articles/ginseng-tea-recipe

Tello, M. (2020, March 25). *Healthy lifestyle: 5 keys to a longer life*. Harvard Health. https://www.health.harvard.edu/blog/healthy-lifestyle-5-keys-to-a-longer-life-2018070514186

Tello, M. (2021, September 14). *Long-lasting healthy changes: Doable and worthwhile*. Harvard Health. https://www.health.harvard.edu/blog/long-lasting-healthy-changes-doable-and-worthwhile-202109142594

13 best natural herbs for sleep. (2022, December 15). Sleep Authority. https://www.sleepauthority.com/sleep-aids/herbs-for-sleep

Thorpe, M., & Amjera, R. (2020, October 27). *12 science-based benefits of meditation*. Healthline. https://www.healthline.com/nutrition/12-benefits-of-meditation

3 herbal tea recipes for wellness. (n.d.). Sips By. https://www.sipsby.com/blogs/tea-recipes/herbal-tea-recipes

Tikkanen, A. (2020). Tea ceremony | description, history, & facts. In *Encyclopædia Britannica*. https://www.britannica.com/topic/tea-ceremony

Top 50 famous tea quotes and tea sayings. (2020, September 21). Simple Loose Leaf Tea Company. https://simplelooseleaf.com/blog/life-with-tea/tea-quotes

Traditional Chinese medicine - herbal therapy. (2019). In *Encyclopædia Britannica*. https://www.britannica.com/science/traditional-Chinese-medicine/Herbal-therapy

Try this peaceful tea meditation to bring comfort to your day. (2020, April 17). Alo

Moves. https://blog.alomoves.com/mindfulness/try-this-peaceful-tea-meditation-to-bring-comfort-to-your-day

The ultimate guide to enjoying a tea ceremony at home. (2021, August 10). Magnifissance. https://magnifissance.com/selfcare/tea/tea-ceremony-at-home/

Understanding the importance of addressing mental health concerns. (n.d.). Her Culture. https://www.herculture.org/blog/2020/9/23/understanding-the-importance-of-addressing-mental-health-concerns

Understanding the stress response. (2020, July 6). Harvard Health. https://www.health.harvard.edu/staying-healthy/understanding-the-stress-response

Van Wyk, B.-E. ., & Gorelik, B. (2017). The history and ethnobotany of Cape herbal teas. *South African Journal of Botany, 110*, 18–38. https://doi.org/10.1016/j.sajb.2016.11.011

Vatel, N. (2020, December 2). *How starting a tea ritual can encourage mindfulness and elevate one's self-care routine.* World Tea News. https://www.worldteanews.com/Features/how-starting-tea-ritual-can-encourage-mindfulness-and-elevate-ones-self-care-routine

Villegas, H. (2022, May 11). *De-stress and relax: An herbal tea recipe to help you manage stress and anxious feelings.* Healing Harvest Homestead. https://healingharvesthomestead.com/home/2017/9/8/de-stress-relax-an-herbal-tea-recipe-to-help-you-out

Villegas, H. (2023, April 11). *How herbs changed my life and health: Why I'll never go back to drugs.* Healing Harvest Homestead. https://healingharvesthomestead.com/home/2019/4/20/how-herbs-transformed-my-health-and-life-plus-why-you-should-learn-about-using-herbs-too

Walters, M. (2022, July 4). *Does tea really help with digestion?* Live Science. https://www.livescience.com/does-tea-really-help-with-digestion

Weight loss: 5 delicious green tea recipes for fat burn. (2022, November 23). *The Times of India.* https://timesofindia.indiatimes.com/life-style/health-fitness/weight-loss/weight-loss-5-delicious-green-tea-recipes-for-fat-burn/photostory/95687369.cms?picid=95687412

Wells, K. (2012, July 11). *10 health boosting herbal teas.* Wellness Mama. https://wellnessmama.com/recipes/health-boosting-herbal-teas

What are anxiety and depression? (2019). Anxiety & Depression Association of America. https://adaa.org/understanding-anxiety

What is anxiety? (2019). Psychology Today. https://www.psychologytoday.com/us/basics/anxiety

What is herbal tea? (2015, October 1). The Republic of Tea. https://www.republicoftea.com/blog/tea-library/what-is-herbal-tea/tl-026/

What meditation can do for your mind, mood, and health. (2014, July 16). Harvard Health. https://www.health.harvard.edu/staying-healthy/what-meditation-can-do-for-your-mind-mood-and-health-

Whelan, C. (2020, September 29). *Can you be allergic to tea?* Healthline. https://www.healthline.com/health/allergies/can-you-be-allergic-to-tea

Worthington, T. (2020, December 16). *Chai tea history: India's favorite drink.* Passion Passport. https://passionpassport.com/chai-tea-history

Your digestive system: 5 ways to support gut health. (n.d.). Johns Hopkins Medicine. https://www.hopkinsmedicine.org/health/wellness-and-prevention/your-digestive-system-5-ways-to-support-gut-health

Your gut instincts: Your guide to digestive wellness. (2013, October 13). Women's Health Network. https://www.womenshealthnetwork.com/digestive-health/natural-digestive-health

Yu, C. (2019, March 24). *How to practice mindfulness with tea.* Senbird Tea. https://senbirdtea.com/how-to-practice-mindfulness-with-tea

Zen. (2022, March 28). *How to make goji berry tea drink (wolfberry tea).* Greedy Girl Gourmet. https://www.greedygirlgourmet.com/how-to-make-goji-berry-tea-drink-wolfberry-tea

IMAGES

Belousova, A. (2019, November 16). *Variety of spices on spoons* [Image]. Pexels. https://www.pexels.com/photo/variety-of-spices-on-spoons-3233275

Bohovyk, O. (2020, January 21). *Clear glass bowl with herbs and tea* [Image]. Pexels. https://www.pexels.com/photo/clear-glass-bowl-with-herbs-and-tea-3604314

Cottonbro Studio. (2020, July 27). *Person holding white and yellow flowers* [Image]. Pexels. https://www.pexels.com/photo/person-holding-white-and-yellow-flowers-4967514

Grabowska, K. (2020, July 14). *Gray mortar and pestle with ground spice* [Image]. Pexels. https://www.pexels.com/photo/gray-mortar-and-pestle-with-ground-spice-4871291

Krukau, Y. (2020, September 29). *Purple flowers on brown wooden table* [Image]. Pexels. https://www.pexels.com/photo/purple-flowers-on-brown-wooden-table-5480238

Leeloo The first. (2021, January 15). *Tea with hibiscus leaves* [Image]. Pexels. https://www.pexels.com/photo/tea-with-hibiscus-leaves-6507025

Mareefe. (2017a, November 6). *Three condiments in plastic containers* [Image]. Pexels. https://www.pexels.com/photo/three-condiments-in-plastic-containers-674483

Mareefe. (2017b, November 7). *Assorted spices near white ceramic bowls* [Image]. Pexels. https://www.pexels.com/photo/assorted-spices-near-white-ceramic-bowls-678414/

Motoc, I. (2020, May 7). *Freshly brewed tea in cup among flowers on windowsill* [Image]. Pexels. https://www.pexels.com/photo/freshly-brewed-tea-in-cup-among-flowers-on-windowsill-4346282

Padriñán, M. Á. (2016, August 1). *Brown wooden spoon with herbs on top of green bamboo mat and brown wooden surface* [Image]. Pexels. https://www.pexels.com/photo/brown-wooden-spoon-with-herbs-on-top-of-green-bamboo-mat-and-brown-wooden-surface-130980

PhotoMIX Company. (2016, May 31). *Purple petaled flowers in mortar and pestle* [Image]. Pexels. https://www.pexels.com/photo/purple-petaled-flowers-in-mortar-and-pestle-105028

Pou, A. (2021a, June 14). *Assorted herbs in bowls* [Image]. Pexels. https://www.pexels.com/photo/assorted-herbs-on-bowls-8330249

Pou, A. (2021b, June 14). *Close up photo of clear glass teapot with herbal tea* [Image]. Pexels. https://www.pexels.com/photo/close-up-photo-of-clear-glass-teapot-with-herbal-tea-8330322

Pou, A. (2021c, June 14). *Close-up of tea in glass teapots* [Image]. Pexels. https://www.pexels.com/photo/clsoe-up-of-tea-in-glass-teapots-8329933

Pou, A. (2021d, June 14). *Herbs and spices on beverage* [Image]. Pexels. https://www.pexels.com/photo/herbs-and-spices-on-beverage-8330390

Pou, A. (2021e, June 14). *Various dried flowers on teaspoons* [Image]. Pexels. https://www.pexels.com/photo/various-dried-flowers-on-teaspoons-8330351

Pou, A. (2021f, June 14). *Woman brewing herb tea and white flowers on table* [Image]. Pexels. https://www.pexels.com/photo/woman-brewing-herb-tea-and-white-flowers-on-table-8329261

Pou, A. (2021g, June 14). *Woman pouring herbal tea into a glass teacup* [Image]. Pexels. https://www.pexels.com/photo/woman-pouring-herbal-tea-into-a-glass-teacup-8329287

Rahmadie, K. (2016, November 11). *Silver round accessory with storage* [Image].

Pexels. https://www.pexels.com/photo/silver-round-accessory-with-storage-227908

Teejay. (2018, August 25). *Clear glass teapot set [Image]*. Pexels. https://www.pexels.com/photo/clear-glass-teapot-set-1362537

ABOUT THE AUTHOR

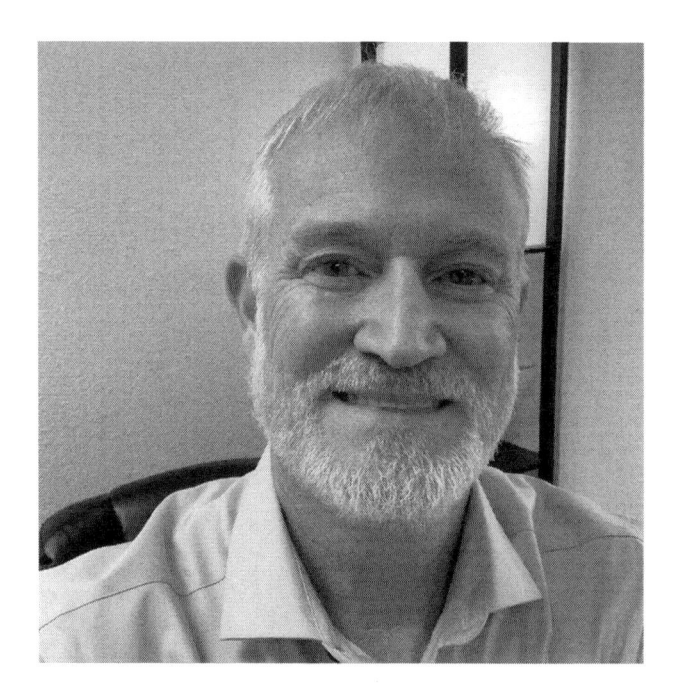

Personal Development Guide Brian Turner is the author of *Herbal Teas Simplified* and *21 Breaths to a Better You*.

Operating in the self-help niche, his writing is devoted to spirituality, philosophy, and alternative health, aiming to deliver a complete approach to holistic wellness and spiritual growth.

Brian has dedicated his life to exploring spirituality and pursuing his personal development. As a certified life coach, he has a strong passion for guiding others on their journeys of physical, emotional, and spiritual wellness. He is a respected teacher and mentor, dedicated to helping others pursue self-discovery, personal growth, and spiritual enlightenment.

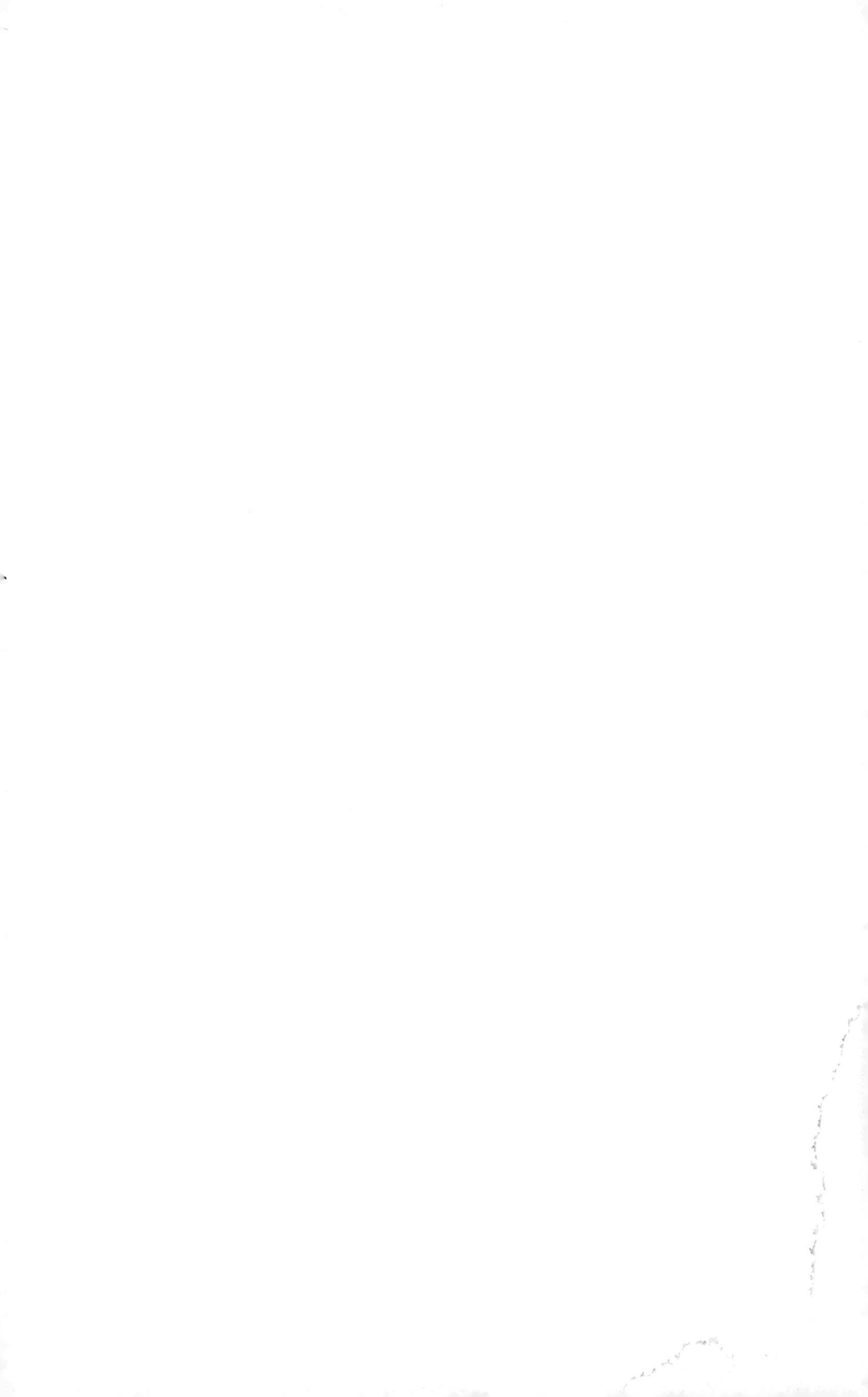

Printed in Great Britain
by Amazon

38711793R00124